Paola Lisset Acevedo Quezada
Aurora Beatriz Ortiz Cruz

Patient care protocol

Paola Lisset Acevedo Quezada
Aurora Beatriz Ortiz Cruz

Patient care protocol

with deep neck abscess of dental origin. A case report

ScienciaScripts

Imprint

Any brand names and product names mentioned in this book are subject to trademark, brand or patent protection and are trademarks or registered trademarks of their respective holders. The use of brand names, product names, common names, trade names, product descriptions etc. even without a particular marking in this work is in no way to be construed to mean that such names may be regarded as unrestricted in respect of trademark and brand protection legislation and could thus be used by anyone.

Cover image: www.ingimage.com

This book is a translation from the original published under ISBN 978-613-9-40129-1.

Publisher:
Sciencia Scripts
is a trademark of
Dodo Books Indian Ocean Ltd. and OmniScriptum S.R.L publishing group

120 High Road, East Finchley, London, N2 9ED, United Kingdom
Str. Armeneasca 28/1, office 1, Chisinau MD-2012, Republic of Moldova, Europe
Printed at: see last page
ISBN: 978-620-7-75964-4

Protocol of care for patients with deep neck abscess of dental origin
in the General Hospital of Xoco: A case report.

Author: *PAOLA LISSET ACEVEDO QUEZADA.
**AURORA BEATRIZ ORTIZ CRUZ.

Table of Contents

INTRODUCTION

Deep neck abscess is a potentially serious clinical entity. Inadequate treatment and management can lead to its progression and be associated with high morbidity and mortality. Deep neck abscess continues to be seen in developing countries such as Mexico.

Odontogenic infections reveal their etiology mainly in periapical lesions, periodontal disease, pulp necrosis, caries as well as bacterial invasion to contiguous anatomical tissues. In terms of microbiology, the most common organisms involved in this infectious process are: Streptococci, Staphylococci, Pepto-streptococci species and anaerobic organisms, constituting a polymicrobial ecosystem.

There are several factors that can influence the complication of the disease such as: age, associated systemic diseases, number and type of anatomical spaces affected. Due to the relationship of the primary aponeurotic spaces with the secondary ones, previously localized odontogenic infections tend to spread rapidly to deep parts of the neck and even proceed to the mediastinum according to the location of the odontogenic infection. It is currently known that infection by deep neck abscess can lead to and predispose to more serious secondary clinical conditions such as airway compromise, mediastinitis, septicemia, systemic inflammatory response syndrome and even necrotizing fasciitis.

Among the most common comorbidities in our Mexican population are endocrinological diseases such as diabetes mellitus, immunodeficiency diseases such as human immunodeficiency virus infection, steroid treatment or cancer patients undergoing chemotherapy or radiotherapy. These patients represent a higher risk of presenting a disease that progresses to severity as well as a greater tendency to develop complications, which is why they should be identified in a timely manner and referred appropriately to minimize the risk of death.

Early impregnation with broad-spectrum intravenous antibiotic treatment, incision, drainage and culture with antibiogram of the secretions (which will provide us with a definitive microbiological study of the causal bacteria), as well as irrigation and continuous manual postoperative surgical cleaning are basic items that are considered the mainstay of treatment for the survival of the patient with deep odontogenic neck infection.

Due to the edema of the mucosa and the anatomical structures involved by the compression generated by the abscess, airway compromise may originate, patients diagnosed with deep neck abscess constantly present airway compromise and this may lead to acute hypoxia. Airway management includes endotracheal intubation or tracheostomy as a treatment strategy.

The main purpose of this work is to inform general dentists, dental specialists and physicians about the etiology, the stages of odontogenic infection and the factors that predispose patients to develop a deep neck abscess, as well as the correct diagnosis of odontogenic abscesses and how to proceed. Always bearing in mind that the main elements in the management of this condition are prevention and timely diagnosis.

HISTORICAL ANTECEDENTS

The first records of the use of drainage in infections were made by Hippocrates of Cos (460-377 B.C.), a physician of ancient Greece, who describes in the Hippocratic treatises, the placement of a drain in the thorax to drain an empyema. [1]

Ambrose Paré (1510-1590), a surgeon of French origin, described the care of wounds and the use of tubes for the drainage of abscesses. The tubes described were made of gold and silver as well as lead and brass; they are dated curved and with holes; he left a tutor thread to avoid the migration of the drain into the abdominal cavity. [2]

In 1543, Andreas Vesalius described that tracheal intubation could save lives.

There is no description of any surgeon before Brasavola (1500-1570) who described the successful surgical treatment of Ludwig's Angina in 1546. [3]

Lorenz Heister (1683-1758), noted anatomist and surgeon of German origin, followed the principle of capillarity in his work Chirurgie, published in 1739, consequently he is also considered one of the promoters and descriptors of capillary drainage, pioneer of drainage by means of Pen rose. [4]

Infection of the facial spaces has been recognized and described since the time of Galen in the 2nd century. Describing a deep cervical space in his studies. A fight against microorganisms by man dates back to ancient civilization. [5]

Odontogenic infections were the fourth leading cause of death according to the London Mortality Acts in the early 17th century, and were associated with a death rate of between 10% and 40% in the pre-antibiotic era. [6]

Ludwig's angina was described around 1836 by the German-born physician Wilhelm Friedrich Von Ludwig. The bacterial cause of the disease was unknown, therefore, Ludwig never related it to an infection and even less odontogenic. He described it as, "A gangrenous induration of the connective tissues involving the muscles of the larynx and the floor of the mouth." He noted that the condition progressively worsened, almost always resulting in death within ten to twelve days. [7]

The origin of the term "antibiotic" goes back to the word antibiosis, which Paul Vuillemin first used as an antonym for symbiosis in his 1890 publication to describe the antagonistic action between different microorganisms. [8]

The later contributions of the German physician Robert Koch were also transformative. His discoveries, including the so-called four "Koch postulates" that establish a causal relationship between microorganisms and disease. [8]

Alexander Fleming, a bacteriologist at St. Mary's Hospital, returned to his laboratory in Paddington (Westminster, London) and found a colony of *Staphylococcus aureus* that he had left on his bench contaminated with a fungus (*Penicillium notatum*). He noticed that, in the vicinity of the mold, the Staphylococci underwent lysis, while colonies farther away appeared normal and unaffected. Fleming cultured and treated several strains of pathogenic bacteria with *Penicillium notatum* to observe effects similar to those previously observed with Staphylococci, especially for Gram positives. He concluded that the fungus excreted a substance that killed the bacteria, and named it penicillin in March 1929.[8]

In the 1930s, Grodinsky and Holyoke described the aponeurotic fasciae and concepts related to the spread of infection through contiguous anatomic spaces. Knowledge of these compartments and their anatomic connection is critical to understanding the spread of head and neck space infections. [9]

In early 1941, policeman Albert Alexander, suffering from a severe facial infection leading to sepsis, was treated with penicillin. His condition improved significantly during the first five days of therapy, but unfortunately the limited supply of drugs ran out and the patient died from the prevailing sepsis. [8]

In the 1943 volume of the Journal of Oral Surgery, Tichy reported on the status of the management of deep neck infections. He ruled that the usual causative bacteria were *Borrelia vincenti*, Streptococcus, Staphylococcus, Diplococcus or *Bacillus septicus*. [6]

In 1945, Fleming pointed out in a New York Times publication about the risk of penicillin due to bacterial resistance (Staphylococcal) and suggested that overuse and underdosage were possibly responsible. [8]

The 1950s would usher in a new crop of novel antibiotics, among the most prominent of which were the erythromycins. [8]

Shortly after the discovery of the erythromycins, another family of antibiotics was discovered, the glycopeptides. The first member of the class was isolated in 1953 from *Streptomyces Orientalis* found in a soil sample from Borneo. Later named vancomycin, it was especially active against Gram-positive bacteria, and against penicillin-resistant Staphylococci. Vancomycin was approved as a clinical agent for the treatment of bacterial infections in 1958. [8]

Pharmaceutical research subsequently altered the chemistry of penicillin, trying to anticipate the rapidly developing resistance, introducing ampicillin to the market, followed by the appearance of amoxicillin, which gave rise to augmentin (amoxicillin with clavulanic acid). [10]

In the 1960s, at Bellevue Hospital, an intramuscular "cocktail" of penicillin and an aminoglycoside (streptomycin) was used without any solid data demonstrating an effective effect in preventing infection in fractured jaws. A few years later, Zallen and Curry reported a controlled study that demonstrated that antibiotics are very effective in preventing postfracture infection. [10]

Trimethoprim is another antibiotic synthesized in 1962, this compound was found to exhibit strong antibacterial activities against Gram-positive and Gram-negative bacteria. In the same year, the first successful clinical data was the discovery of synergistic effects when the drug was administered to patients together with sulfonamides. [8]

Prior to the 1980s, the decision to hospitalize patients with odontogenic infections was a hotly debated topic, based on experience and surgical judgment. [10]

Numerous generations of cephalosporins are currently available, as well as lincomycin, which gave rise to clindamycin, and other options such as macrolides and fluoroquinolones. [10]

CELLULITIS

It is defined as that phase that occurs in the course of the development of an undemarcated odontogenic infection in which there is absence of pus and occurs after 3-5 days, where the inflammation becomes firmer, red and very painful on palpation, resulting from the infecting mixed flora that stimulates the intense inflammatory response. [11]

ABSCESO

An abscess is defined as a localized collection of pus in a cavity formed as a consequence of cellular decomposition and tissue necrosis (pyogenic membrane), resulting in a firm, painful and fluctuating erythematous nodule. [12]

ETIOPATHOGENY

Most of the time, the bacteria involved in the infectious process are part of the commensal flora that normally inhabits the host's native environment, and when an imbalance is generated between the host and the causative agent, the infection occurs. These bacteria are mostly Gram-positive aerobic cocci, Gram-positive anaerobic cocci and finally Gram-negative anaerobic bacilli, which are the main causes of several common ailments, such as dental caries, gingivitis and periodontitis. When these bacteria manage to penetrate into the underlying deep tissues, for example, in a tooth with necrotic dental pulp or from a periodontal pocket, there is a high possibility of originating an odontogenic infection. [11]

Odontogenic infections take their origin mainly from two well described locations:

> 1) Periapical localization, as a result of pulp necrosis and consequent bacterial penetration into the periapical tissues.

> 2) Periodontal location, as a result of the formation of a deep periodontal pocket that enables the inoculation of bacteria to the surrounding soft tissues.

From these two origins, the apical origin is the most common in the development of odontogenic infections.[11]

Pulp necrosis takes its etiology from an untreated deep caries, which provides a perfect entry route for bacteria to penetrate the periapical tissues. After being inoculated into these tissues and establishing a potentially active infection, the infection tends to spread in all possible paths. The infection spreads by following the path into the cancellous bone until it encounters a cortical plate of bone. If this cortical plate is thin, the infection succeeds in eroding the entire bone and thereby penetrating the surrounding soft tissues. [11]

As the infection continues to progress to deeper levels, different members of the infecting flora have the ability to find ideal conditions for development and therefore increase in number based on other species previously dominant in the environment. The polymicrobial and multimicrobial condition of these infections makes it extremely important for the clinician to assimilate and identify the great variety of bacteria that are probably the cause of the infection. In most odontogenic infections, an average of five species of bacteria can be identified developing at the same time in the acute process, analyzed by culture. [11]

Another extremely important factor is the oxygen tolerance capacity of bacteria in odontogenic infections. The oral flora is a conjugation of bacteria of aerobic and anaerobic origin, it is common to detect that in most odontogenic infections these two types of bacteria are present. Infections originating solely from bacteria of aerobic origin are specifically considered to account for 6% of all odontogenic infections. Anaerobic bacteria are found in 44% of these infections. Odontogenic infections caused by a confluence of aerobic and anaerobic bacteria account for 50% of all odontogenic infections. [11]

The dominant bacteria of aerobic origin in odontogenic infections are those corresponding to the group of: *Streptococcus milleri, S. viridans: S. anginosus, S. intermedius and S. constellatus.* These facultative bacteria are able to develop in the presence as well as in the absence of oxygen, having the ability to initiate the process of invasion into deeper tissues. [11]

The mechanism by which this mixed bacterial flora produces and develops infection is now precisely understood. After the first step, which is bacterial inoculation into the deep tissues, the facultative microorganisms of the *S. milleri* group begin to synthesize hyaluronidase, which allows the dissemination and spread and invasion of the bacteria causing the infection, taking its way through the connective tissue that will subsequently lead to the onset of the clinical presentation known as: Cellulitic stage of odontogenic infection. [11]

The metabolic by-products produced by the Streptococcus group provide a favorable environment for the growth and development of anaerobic microorganisms, which are:

1. Release of essential nutrients.

2. A low tissue pH.

3. Consumption of local oxygen supply. [11]

In this environment, bacteria of aerobic origin can develop and predominate and, as the oxygen-reduction potential is reduced, bacteria of anaerobic origin begin to predominate, which have the capacity to cause necrosis and tissue liquefaction thanks to the synthesis of collagenase-type proteins. With the degradation of collagen and in conjunction with necrosis and lysis of the leukocytes present in the infection, a stage of formation of microabscesses is achieved which tend to fuse until a well-demarcated abscess with clinically recognizable signs is generated. In the abscess stage, bacteria of anaerobic origin are mostly identified and, on some occasions, they may be the only microorganisms identified in microbiological cultures. [11]

The evolution from an aerobic to an anaerobic flora is related to the type of inflammation that occurs in the infected area. Therefore, odontogenic infections are studied and described in four phases:

1. In the first 3 days of symptom onset, a pasty type inflammation with a soft consistency and slightly painful to palpation is described, which represents the inoculation phase, in which Streptococci begin to form colonies and invade the host.

2. Between days 3-5, the inflammation becomes more firm and consolidated, with a red appearance and painful to palpation, at this stage the mixed bacterial flora stimulates an intense inflammatory response which is known as the cellulite phase or cellulite phase.

3. Between days 5 and 7 anaerobic microorganisms begin to prevail, which produce an abscess described as "liquefaction" type, in the central zone of the inflamed and infected area. This phase is known as the abscess phase. The yellow color of the underlying pus can be seen through the thin epithelial layers. At this stage the term fluctuation is appropriately applied. Fluctuation involves palpation of a wave of fluid with one hand while the abscess is compressed with the other.

4. Finally, if the abscess has an outcome whereby it drains spontaneously through the skin, mucosa or is surgically drained, the resolution phase begins, characterized by a rise in the immune system, which begins to fight the bacteria causing the infection, followed by a process of healing and tissue repair. [11, 12]

When infection erodes the cortical plate of the alveolar aspect of the bone it spreads to predictable anatomical locations. The location of the infection arising from a specific tooth is determined by two main factors: the thickness of the bone surrounding the apex of the tooth and the relationship of the bone perforation zone to the muscular insertions of the facial mass. [11]

See table n.1 Description of the stages and evolution of odontogenic infection. [11]

Stages and evolution of odontogenic infection.			
Features	Inoculation time (edema)	Cellulite	Abscess

Duration	0 - 3 days	3-7 days	After 5 days
Pain scale	Medium-moderate	Severe and generalized	Severe-moderate and localized
Size	Variable	Grande	Menor
Location	Fuzzy	Fuzzy	Circumscribed
Palpation	Soft, doughy, gelatinous	Indurada	Fluctuating, softer center
Appearance	Normal coloring	Erythematous	Erythematous in the periphery
Clinical features	Normal	Woody	Bright center
Temperature of the area	Normal or mild hyperemia	Mild hyperemia	Moderately hyperemic
Loss of function	Normal or minimum	Severa	Moderately severe
Degree of discomfort	Edema	Hematic content, pus	Pus
Gravity	Medium	Severo	Moderately severe
Progression	On the rise	Growing	Decreasing

Predominant bacteria	Aerobic	Mixed	Anaerobic

CERVICAL FASCIAE

Fascia is defined as an enveloping and surrounding sheet of dense fibrous connective tissue located beneath the skin. There are different layers that protect and envelop the muscle tissue either of superficial origin or with a deeper origin. [9]

The superficial fascia is a layer composed of connective tissue located immediately beneath the skin. It contains fat, blood vessels, lymphatics, glands and nerves. [9]

Deep fascia, also known as investing fascia, wraps around muscles and serves to support tissues as an elastic sheath. It can provide fibrous sheaths for tendons, muscle origins and insertions, and the formation of retinaculae. (The word "retinaculum" comes from the Latin *retinaculum* and means "web-like structure that gives support to an organ or tissue"). [9]

The deep cervical fascia is composed of three layers: superficial layer, middle layer and deep layer. [9]

The superficial layer, also known as the lining layer, surrounds the trapezius muscle, the sternocleidomastoid muscle, the submandibular gland and the parotid gland. Superiorly, this layer is contiguous with the deep temporalis fascia and the parotid-maseteric fascia. [9]

The middle layer consists of a fascia that surrounds the infrahyoid muscles and has two layers that envelop the sternohyoid, omohyoid, sternothyroid and thyrohyoid structures. [9]

The visceral fascia envelops the thyroid, trachea, larynx, esophagus and pharynx.

The buccopharyngeal fascia covers the buccinator muscle and pharynx to fuse with the pretracheal fascia. [9]

The pretracheal fascia lines the thyroid gland, trachea and larynx and fuses to the inferior part of the pericardium. [9]

The deep layer is formed by the alar and prevertebral fascia. The alar fascia separates from the prevertebral fascia to pass between the vertebral transverse processes and joins the carotid sheath laterally. The prevertebral fascia is a sheath that encloses the vertebral column and its muscles. It contains axillary vessels, brachial plexus and sympathetic trunks. [9]

Infections have the capacity to affect structures contiguous and close to the mediastinum taking their origin from the retropharyngeal, pretracheal and prevertebral spaces. [9]

The carotid sheath is a structure composed of layers of deep cervical fascia; it contains the vagus nerve, the internal jugular vein and the common and internal carotid arteries. [9]

Eleven "aponeurotic spaces" created by the fasciae are known to be present and in contiguity with the deep anatomy of the neck. [9]

APONEUROTIC SPACES

Potentially dangerous aponeurotic spaces of the neck are described based on a complex anatomy where infections are often secondary to contiguous spread from local sites, which continue along facial planes to ultimately create abscesses and/or penetration of infection into the deep neck space level. [13]

***See table n.2 (Classification of the anatomical spaces of the head and neck according to their level of severity in the course of an odontogenic infection).* [11]**

The primary odontogenic aponeurotic spaces involve facial spaces that are in direct association and relationship with the dentoalveolar complex. The dentoalveolar complex is composed of the teeth, gingival tissues and surrounding bone tissue. [9]

A primary odontogenic aponeurotic space is directly contiguous to the origin of the dentoalveolar odontogenic infection. They are classified into: Infraorbital, Buccal, Subperiosteal, Infratemporal, Superficial Temporal, Submandibular, Submentonian, Sublingual, Pterygomandibular, Submaseteric. [9]

A secondary odontogenic aponeurotic space is close to a primary space and may be affected due to anatomical association. They are classified into: Lateral pharyngeal, Retropharyngeal, Parotid, Prevertebral, Pretracheal, Danger space, Carotid space.[9]

Classification of head and neck anatomical spaces according to their severity.	
Severity grade 1: Low degree of threat to vital anatomical structures.	Vestibular Subperiosteal Infraorbital Oral

Severity grade 2: Average severity of threat to vital anatomical structures.	Submandibular Submental Sublingual Pterygomandibular Submasseteric Temporary superficial Deep temporal (infratemporal)
Severity grade 3: High severity of threat to vital anatomical structures.	Lateral pharyngeal Retropharyngeal Pretracheal
Severity grade 4: Extreme severity of threat to vital anatomical structures.	Danger space Mediastinum Intracranial infection

DISSEMINATION AND ANATOMIC DRAINAGE

Table 3 lists the tendency for infectious dissemination according to the tooth involved, as well as the content, anatomical relationships and type of approach recommended for incision and drainage of each anatomical space. [14]

Relationships, contents and approaches in deep aponeurotic spaces.				
Space	Common causes and related teeth	Content	Adjacent spaces	Type of approach recommended for incision and drainage
Oral	Upper molars Lower molars	Parotid duct Anterior facial artery and vein Transverse facial artery and vein Oral fat	Infraorbital Pterygomandibular Infratemporal	Intraoral (small) Extraoral (wide)
Infraorbital	Upper molars, upper canines	Angular artery and vein Infraorbital nerve	Oral	Intraoral
Submandibular	Lower molars	Submandibular gland Facial artery and vein Lymph nodes	Sublingual Submental Lateral pharyngeal Oral	Extraoral
Submental	Previous lower	Anterior jugular vein	Submandibular	Extraoral

	Fracture of the mandibular symphysis	Lymph nodes		
Sublingual	Lower molars Direct trauma	Sublingual gland Wharton duct Lingual nerve Sublingual artery and vein	Submandibular Lateral pharyngeal Visceral (trachea, esophagus)	Intraoral Intraoral - Extraoral
Pterygomandibular	Lower third molars Mandibular angle fracture	Mandibular division of the trigeminal n. Inferior alveolar artery and vein	Oral Lateral pharyngeal Submaseteric Deep temporary Parotideo Peritonsillar	Intraoral Intraoral - Extraoral
Submaseteric	Lower third molars Mandibular angle fracture	Masseteric artery and vein	Oral Pterygomandibular Temporary superficial Parotideo	Intraoral Intraoral - Extraoral
Infratemporal and deep temporal	Upper molars	Pterygoid plexus Maxillary artery and vein Mandibular division of the trigeminal n.	Oral Temporary superficial Inferior petrosal sinus (venous)	Intraoral Extraoral Intraoral - Extraoral

Temporary superficial	Upper molars Lower molars	Temporary grease Temporal branch of the facial n.	Oral Deep temporary	Intraoral Extraoral Intraoral - Extraoral
Lateral pharyngeal or parapharyngeal	Lower third molars Tonsillar infection in contiguous spaces	Carotid artery Internal jugular vein Vagus nerve Cervical sympathetic chain	Pterygomandibular Submandibular Sublingual Peritonsillar Retropharyngeal	Intraoral Intraoral - Extraoral

Table 4 shows the borders and limits of each of the deep anatomical spaces of the head and neck. [14]

Space	Front edge	Rear edge	Top edge	Bottom edge	Superficial or medial	Deep or lateral
Oral	Labial commissure	Masseter muscle	Maxilla Infraorbital space	Skin and jaw tissue	Subcutaneous tissue	Buccinator muscle

Infraorbital	Nasal cartilages	Buccal space	Levator labii superioris muscle	Oral mucosa Levator anguli oris muscle	Levator labii superioris muscle	Levator anguli oris muscle, maxillary
Submandibular	Anterior belly of the digastric muscle	Posterior belly of digastric, stylohyoid, stylopharyngeus pharyngeus muscles	Inferior and medial surface of the mandible	Tendon of the digastric muscle	Platysma and enveloping fascia muscle	Mylohyoid, hyoglossus and upper constrictor muscles
Submental	Mandibular lower border	Hyoid bone	Mylohyohyoid muscle			Anterior bellies of the digastric muscle
Sublingual	Mandibular lingual surface	Submandibular space	Oral mucosa	Mylohyohyoid muscle	Muscles of the tongue	Lingual surface of the mandible
Pterygomandibular	Buccal space	Parotid gland	Lateral pterygoid muscle	Mandibular lower border	Medial pterygogoid muscle	Mandibular ascending branches

Submasseteric	Buccal space	Parotid gland	Zygomatic arch	Mandibular lower border	Mandibular ascending branch	Masseter muscle
Lateral pharyngeal	Upper and middle pharyngeal constrictor muscles	Carotid sheath and scalene fascia	Base of skull	Hyoid bone	Pharyngeal constrictors and retropharyngeal space	Medial pterygoid muscle
Retropharyngeal	Upper and middle pharyngeal constrictor muscles	Wing fascia	Base of skull	Fusion of the alar and prevertebral fascia at the cervical 6 and thoracic 4 level.	-	Carotid vena cava and lateral pharyngeal space
Pretracheal	Sternothyroid and thyrohyoid fascia	Retropharyngeal space	Thyroid cartilage	Upper mediastinum	Sternothyroid - thyrohyoid fascia	Visceral fascia, trachea, thyroid gland

Odontogenic infections that take their origin from infected/carious lower molars tend to destroy the cortical bone of the lingual area more frequently. Infections of molars take their drainage path either buccally or lingually. The mylohyoid muscle is an anatomical point of utmost relevance as it determines whether the odontogenic infection that drained lingually will progress to limits above this muscle in the sublingual space or below it at the level of the submandibular plane.[11]

The odontogenic infection that frequently prevails is the abscess of the vestibular space. Very often, patients do not seek any treatment for this condition and it goes unnoticed, as a consequence the condition may drain spontaneously, which will generate its resolution or on the other hand the chronicity of the condition. The infection tends to reappear due to a closure of the previously drained area. Sometimes the abscess creates a chronic sinuous tract that drains into the oral cavity or skin. As long as the chronic sinuous tract continues to drain, the patient will not suffer pain; however, this would be the ideal scenario, but not the frequent one, much less the solution to the problem. Usually, the administration of antibiotics temporarily stops the drainage of infected material, but at the end of the antibiotic cycle the suppuration reappears due to the failure to remove or treat the septic focus. [11]

TREATMENT RATIONALE/PROTOCOL:

The number one step in admitting the patient to the hospital is medical propaedeutics, as well as timely diagnosis, the surgeon must have the judgment to assess the rate of progression and evolution of the condition by asking about the onset of symptoms such as swelling (increase in volume), pain, temperature, consistency, trismus and airway involvement. Author Flynn and colleagues found that the number of days of swelling prior to the patient's admission to the hospital correlates negatively with the estimate of initial severity. [11,14]

The eight steps in the management of odontogenic infections are listed and discussed as follows:

1. Determine the severity of the infection.
2. Assess host defenses.
3. Decide the scope of medical care (outpatient/inpatient).
4. Treat surgically.
5. Medical support.
6. Choose and prescribe antimicrobial therapy.
7. Administer the antibiotic correctly.
8. Evaluate the patient frequently. [14]

Rationale 1: Determine severity of infection.

1. Take a complete medical history:

- The initial purpose is to find out the patient's initial symptom and its evolution time.
- The symptoms should be written in the same words as those referred by the patient.
- It should be stipulated:

a) How many days of evolution has the odontogenic infection been active since the patient noticed the first symptom.

b) Determine the course of the odontogenic infection: the patient reports relapses, worsening, stabilization, improvement.

c) Determine how fast the infectious process has spread.

d) Describe the patient's symptoms: flushing, tumor, pain, heat, loss of function.

e) Determine the general condition of the patient: febrile, weak, asthenia, adynamia, hyperthermia, hypothermia, loss of appetite, dysphagia, odynophagia, tachypnea, bradypnea, tachycardia, bradycardia, oliguria, etc. [11]

2. Physical examination:

a. It is necessary to assess vital signs: temperature, heart rate, blood pressure, respiratory rate, oxygen saturation.

b. If the heart rate is above 100 beats/min, the patient may have a serious infection and needs to be treated more vigorously.

c. The vital sign that varies the least with infection is blood pressure.

d. Only if the patient is in severe pain and anxiety will there be an elevation of systolic blood pressure. However, it is important to note that septic shock causes hypotension. [11]

See table n. 5, Diagnostic criteria presented in Systemic Inflammatory Response Syndrome. [15]

See table n. 6, Criteria for hospital admission in patients with deep neck abscess. [15]

3. Palpation and inspection

Areas subject to inflammation should be explored by palpation.

The surgeon will palpate the area of inflammation in search of any discomfort such as increased local heat in the area and the consistency of the swollen area, this can vary from being perceived as soft and similar to normal to show as a firm, fleshy (pasty) or even hard (indurated) inflammation. An indurated swelling has a firmness comparable to that of a contracting muscle.

Another consistency that can be found is fluctuating. Fluctuant is defined and compared as the sensation of a fluid-filled balloon. Fluctuant presentations most often indicate the accumulation of liquid pus in the center of an indurated area. *See figure n.*1 [11]

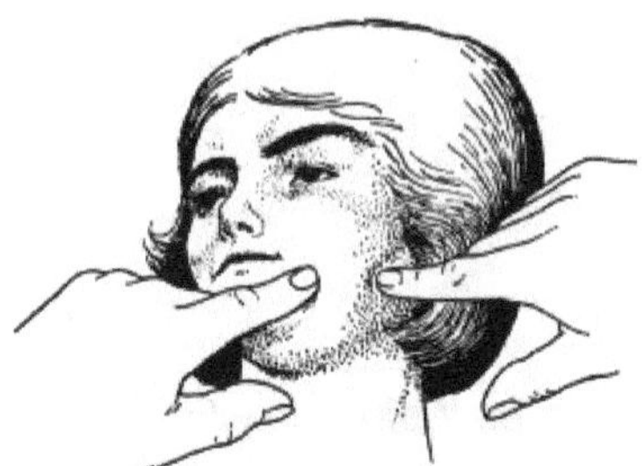

Fig. n. 1 Exemplification of the palpation method for fluctuation. [24]

The surgeon must perform an intraoral exploration in search of the specific cause also known as septic focus of infection. There may be the presence of teeth in poor condition such as deep and advanced caries, an abscess of periodontal origin, periodontal disease, combinations of caries and periodontal disease or a fracture in the process of infection. [11]

See table n. 5, Diagnostic criteria presented in Systemic Inflammatory Response Syndrome. 15

Diagnostic criteria in Systemic Inflammatory Response Syndrome (SIRS).
If 2 or more of the following conditions are present:
•   Temperature <36° or >38°.
•   Pulse > 90 beats/min.
•   Respiratory rate >20 resp/min.
•   Blood pressure < 32 mm Hg.
•   Leukocyte count <4000 cells/mm^3 or > 12,000 cells/ mm^3 .

See table n. 6, Criteria for hospital admission in patients with deep neck abscess. 15

Criteria for hospital admission.
§ Temperature >38°.

§ Dehydration.
§ Compromised airway or vital structures.
§ Infection in anatomical spaces of moderate or severe severity.
§ Need for general anesthesia.
§ Systemic decontrol.

<u>Imaging evaluation</u>

Diagnostic imaging plays a fundamental role in the diagnosis of pathologies in head and neck infections. It is crucial that the surgeon has an adequate knowledge of the anatomy of the head and neck as well as each of the spaces and contents of the neck, recognizing the different boundaries and anatomical structures that contain each one, the knowledge of this information provides the optimal understanding for an adequate diagnosis of the current condition to which the patient is being subjected in clinical practice. [16]

Computed tomography was created by Hounsfield and Cormack, who were awarded the Nobel Prize in Physiology and Medicine in 1979. Computed tomography images are a computer-generated digitization of multiple radiographs and slices obtained when the source and detector rotate around the patient under study. [17]

The information is then transformed using complex formulas and mechanisms based on voxel units. A voxel is the cubic unit that makes up a three-dimensional object. [17]

The relative radiodensity of each voxel is given a numerical value known as a Hounsfield unit (HU), where the relative absorption of X-ray energy is quantified in comparison to water. Some common HU values for reference are air (-1000 HU), fat (-100 to -80 HU), water (0 HU), blood (60 to 110 HU) and bone (1000 HU). [17]

However, computed tomography (CT), magnetic resonance imaging (MRI) or Cone Beam should be necessary for a reliable assessment of the extent of infection to deeper and surrounding structures. CT is especially useful for the evaluation of acute inflammatory processes because it has the ability to depict and show erosion and destruction of cortical bone, as well as soft tissue window and even used as a contrast medium, it also allows the observation of calculi (e.g., submandibular duct). [18]

Correct and reliable imaging interpretation requires a broad knowledge of human anatomy, as well as knowledge of the variations in anatomical structures that may occur and the changes caused by pathology or infection. [19]

Usually, the anatomy of the facial and skull mass on a CT scan can be studied by means of sagittal, coronal, axial or transverse slices and 3D three-dimensional reconstructions. [19]

The imaging anatomy of the facial mass and skull is studied systematically. Its study can be performed by two common methods: analyzing the sections from its caudal to cephalic origin (inferior to superior), and the anatomy of the neck is studied from its cephalic to caudal origin. [19]

<u>Axial cuts</u>

The maxillofacial bone anatomy begins with the identification of the hyoid bone, the epiglottis and the pharyngeal airway together with the mandibular symphysis, observing at this level the fourth cervical vertebra. At a more cephalic level, the mandible is observed in more detail. The third cervical vertebra is at this level. Superiorly, the odontoid process of the second cervical vertebra is observed, circumscribed by the anterior and posterior arches of the atlas.

The mandibular foramen can also be seen. Looking cephalad, the bilateral mandibular branches can be seen; at this level the mastoid air cells and the foramen magnum can be seen. [19]

Continuing in the cephalic direction, the maxillary sinuses can be clearly seen along with the zygomatic arches. The condyles are clearly visible at this level.

The nasal anatomy can be seen starting from the floor of the nostrils. Superiorly, slices show the nasolacrimal ducts, and the floor of the sphenoid sinus.

Further cephalic slices from this point expose the uppermost portions of the inferior orbital fissure, middle cranial fossa and posterior cranial fossa. A superior slice shows the frontal sinuses and crista galli, as well as the parietal bones. [19]

<u>Coronal slices</u>

The anatomical areas of importance start from the anterior aspect of the mandibular bone, the maxillary bone, the orbits and the frontal bone. The mentonian symphysis is seen in conjunction with the anterior teeth and in this vertical or coronal plane the anterior portions of the maxillary sinuses can be observed, as well as the nasal anatomy, the ethmoidal cells, the two orbits and the frontal sinuses.

Addressing posteriorly, the isodensity of the tongue and the bony anatomy of the bilateral mandible along with the mentonian foramen or also known as the inferior alveolar nerve canal at bilateral, the maxillary sinuses along with the nasal septum, the bilateral nasal turbinates (inferior and middle), the unciform process of the ethmoid, the ethmoidal air cells, the lamina cribrosa of the ethmoid, the crista galli and the frontal bone can be identified. [19]

Subsequently, the zygomaticofrontal suture, the zygomaticofacial foramen and, in the mandibular bone, the fossa housing the submandibular gland can be examined.

The sphenoid air cells, the pterygoid laminae (medial and lateral) of the sphenoid, the vomer bone, the bilateral mandibular branches are visualized posteriorly.

As the airspace corresponding to the pharynx is studied, an anatomical structure known as Rosenmüller's fossa can be examined. This is a deep, shallow, narrow depression located in the farthest section of the nasal cavity. It is located behind the ostium. [19]

At this level, the foramen rotundum (greater round foramen) can be seen. The greater round foramen gives way to the maxillary branch V2 of the trigeminal nerve.
The greater palatine foramen can be identified in the posterior part corresponding to the hard palate.

Towards the posterior wall of the pharyngeal air space, we will have as bony landmarks the hyoid bone, the anterior arch of cervical vertebra 1, the clivus and the bilateral mandibular condyles together with their glenoid cavities and the visualization of the middle cranial fossa in this location. [19]

<u>Sagittal slices</u>

Because the anatomy is the same in both hemifaces, not always symmetrical anatomy in a sagittal slice can be studied by comparing and controlling one side of the hemiface with the other. Starting from the mid-sagittal plane in the midline, structures including soft and bony tissues can be easily identified by this slice.

The mandibular bone, the geni processes, the incisive foramen in the maxillary bone, the lingual foramen in the mandibular bone, the hard palate, the soft palate, the epiglottis, the anterior nasal spine, the posterior nasal spine, the uvula, the nasal bones, the sphenoid sinuses, the frontal sinuses, the dorsum of the sella turcica, the clivus, the anterior and posterior arches of the atlas, are some of the anatomical structures, the nasal bones, the sphenoid sinuses, the frontal sinuses, the dorsum of the sella turcica, the clivus, the anterior and posterior arches of the atlas, are some of the anatomical structures that can be observed in this section. [19]

The posterior pharyngeal wall can be seen more clearly in this section, laterally, the nasal turbinates can be identified together with the rest of the palate, the ethmoidal sinuses and the lateral part of the pharyngeal airway. Some parts of the cervical vertebrae can be observed but not a complete anatomical study of them. A more lateral view gives us the view of the unilateral mandibular condyles, the corresponding glenoid cavities, the external auditory meatus, the articular eminence and the mastoid process. [19]

Maximum intensity projections (MIP) are image reconstructions based on a rendering method, which secondarily provides tomographic data and slices necessary to form a 3-D image that projects the maximum intensity voxels onto the visual plane. This technique was invented by Wallis and colleagues in 1989. [18]

In maxillofacial imaging, this technique is of great importance because it is possible to reconstruct the image three-dimensionally and observe the anatomical structures from multiple viewing angles of the physician's choice, obtaining a broad understanding of the situation. [18]

3-D reconstructions are part of the display in most software applications and Digital Imaging and Communication in Medicine (DICOM) viewers. The reconstruction algorithms allow an accurate depiction of the bony anatomy. [18]

4. Airway compromise:

One of the fundamental considerations in odontogenic infections is the high prevalence of either partial or complete airway obstruction as an inference of the extension of the infection to deep neck planes.

Careful observation should be made to ensure that the airway is clear and that the patient can breathe without any difficulty. The normal respiratory rate is 14 to 16 breaths per minute (resp/min). Patients with infections classified as mild to moderate may have elevated respiratory rates above 18 resp/min. Oxygen saturation below 94% indicates insufficient tissue oxygenation due to hypoperfusion or hypooxygenation. [11]

The most common leading cause of death in diagnoses reported as odontogenic infection is upper airway obstruction. Therefore, the surgeon should evaluate and estimate the presence of current or impending airway obstruction early in the clinical evaluation of the patient in the course of a severe odontogenic infection. [11]

Complete airway obstruction is a hospital surgical emergency. In the case of partial airway obstruction, the presence of abnormal breath sounds will be noticeable, residing in stridor and wheezing, and may suggest the presence of fluid/pus in the upper airway. [11]
The patient may adopt a very noticeable posture which is intended to straighten the airway, similar to the *sniffing position*, in which the head is tilted forward and the chin is raised, as if sniffing some object. [11]

Another posture indicative of this condition may occur in the patient sitting with his hands or elbows placed on his knees and with the chest tilted forward pushing the head in front of the shoulders, which is intended to straighten the airway and allow accumulated secretions to exit toward the floor. Eventually, a patient with an odontogenic infection occupying the lateral pharyngeal space will often tilt the neck toward the shoulder opposite the affected side. [11]

A crucial point is to evaluate the position of the uvula, as well as the state of the anterior tonsillar pillars. The affected tonsillar pillar is usually edematous and reddened, displacing the uvula to the opposite side of the affected one. **See figure n.2**

If the suspected site of infection is touched with the mirror or tongue depressor, sharp pain may occur, particularly in comparison to the opposite unaffected side. [11]

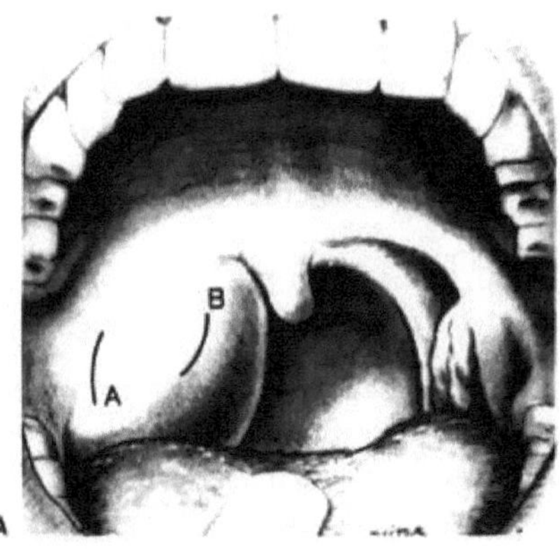

Fig. n. 2 Illustration showing involvement of the lateral pharyngeal space as well as the anterior tonsillar pillars.

A) Incision for drainage of lateral pharyngeal space

B) Incision for drainage of the masseteric and pterygoid space. [24]

Currently, several clinical and methodical tests have been proposed in order to predict difficult intubation, such as the Mallampati test. [13]

Soft tissue radiographs as well as cervical airway and chest radiographs are very valuable in identifying lateral airway deviation, anterior or posterior displacement of the airway on a lateral projection, posteroanterior radiograph or computed tomography. These diagnostic methods are advantageous for the radiographic evaluation of the patient with significant cervical swelling. [13]

To maximize patient safety, it is reasonable to attempt to predict a difficult airway and adjust airway management accordingly. Comprehensive airway assessment includes consideration of each individual's anatomic and physiologic characteristics, as well as contextual issues that may affect the approach to airway management (e.g., Ludwig angina). However, airway examination is only one aspect of difficult airway management. The other aspects are skills, techniques and factors related to the physician in question. [20]

Predictors of airway management difficulty can be classified into:

Anatomical factors.

2. Physiological or contextual factors. [20]

Anatomic predictors can be divided into predictors of difficult direct or video laryngoscopy, difficult face mask ventilation, difficult insertion or use of the supraglottic airway, and difficult access to the frontal neck airway. [20]

Obese patients are twice as likely to have a severe airway complication, patients with a body mass index greater than 40 (morbid obesity) are 4 times more likely to have a severe intubation complication. [20]

The anatomical changes that accompany obesity are: a neck circumference of more than 40 cm, which are associated with difficulty in mask ventilation, difficulty in laryngoscopy and difficulty in tracheal intubation. Obesity or a thick neck also predicts difficult identification of landmarks for cricothyrotomy and tracheostomy. [20]

Rationale 2: Assess host defenses.

The objective of this evaluation is to predict the host's defense capacity against infection. Different conditions and comorbidities are known to make it difficult for both humoral and cellular defenses to perform their functions fully or as they should. There are a number of specific diseases which may contribute to lowering host defenses. [11]

According to the author Ellis Hupp classifies these predisposing conditions as follows:

1.- Uncontrolled metabolic diseases: poorly controlled diabetes, alcoholism, malnutrition, end-stage renal failure.

Immunosuppressive diseases: human immunodeficiency virus, lymphomas, leukemias, oncologic processes, congenital and acquired immunologic diseases.

Immunosuppressive treatments: anticancer chemotherapy, corticosteroids, organ transplantation. Anticancer chemotherapy drugs can decrease the total number of circulating leukocytes to very low numbers, usually less than 1,000 cells per milliliter (cell/ml). [11]

In several studies reported according to the author Petterson in his second edition of the book Principles of Oral and Maxillofacial Surgery, he tells us that the white blood cell count on admission of the patient to the hospital unit has been a significant predictor of the length of the patient's hospital stay. Consequently, the continuous evaluation of leukocytosis or leukopenia is an important and determining factor in the severity of the odontogenic infection which can estimate the duration and evolution of the hospital stay. [14]

C-reactive protein (CRP) is known as an acute phase protein and can be quantified in plasma after it has been synthesized in hepatocytes. The initial trigger for CRP production is the release of interleukin-1 by macrophages near the affected tissue site. [21]

CRP is related to the innate immune system and therefore activates neutrophils, participating in the eradication of antigens and activating the complement system.

CRP can be measured in the serum of healthy people with a level of 0-3 mg/L. After any inflammatory process, CRP levels increase within a few hours. [21]

Leukocytes have a life span of 5 to 6 days; hence the origin of the fact that the progression of the infection is more accurately represented by CRP quantified within a few hours of the onset of acute illness. Leukocytes in the serum of healthy persons range from 4,000 to 11,000 thousand cells per mm3. By producing, transporting and distributing antibodies as part of the immune system, the number of leukocytes increases in response to infection and inflammation processes. [21]

After being synthesized in the liver, CRP levels increase within a few hours after the onset of symptoms and peak at 24-48 h.

Once the inflammatory processes are resolved, CRP levels decrease in a short period of time, due to the short life of the molecules (5-7 hours).

The rapid rise and fall of CRP levels in acute inflammatory processes makes these levels a more sensitive indicator of infection than even erythrocyte sedimentation rate (ESR) or white blood cell count. [21]

Rationale 3: Decide whether the management of the patient should be carried out by the general dentist or the maxillofacial surgeon specialist.

When a patient with a diagnosis of odontogenic infection comes to the dental office for treatment, the dental practitioner should rely on a set of criteria established in the natural disease history of this condition in order to determine the severity of the odontogenic infection. If some or all of these parameters are met, immediate transfer of the patient to a specialist and hospital should certainly be considered. [11]

There are currently three main criteria that indicate the need for immediate referral to a hospital emergency department because it poses an imminent threat to the patient's life and airway:

1.- A history of rapidly evolving infection is known. This would mean that the infection originated 1 or 2 days before the consultation and that it is worsening very rapidly, presenting with increased volume, pain and other associated signs and symptoms.

The second criterion is shortness of breath (dyspnea). Patients who, as a consequence of the infection, manifest an intense inflammation of the soft tissues, as well as of the upper respiratory tract, may have difficulty in keeping the upper airway permeable.

The third and last emergency criterion is difficulty in swallowing (dysphagia). The dribbling of saliva, also known as drooling, is a fundamental sign since it shows the inability to control the patient's own secretions, which frequently indicates the existence of a narrowing at the level of the oropharynx and the possibility of acute obstruction of the upper airway. [11]

Odontogenic infections that spread beyond the limits of the mandibular bone pose a strong threat to the upper respiratory tract and these have the propensity to cause deep neck infections. [22]

Serious complications have been reported including brain abscess, descending mediastinitis, toxic shock syndrome, necrotizing fasciitis, and the development of methicillin-resistant *Staphylococcus aureus* (MRSA) while in the ICU (Intensive Care Unit). [22]

Rationale 4: Treat infection surgically.

The purpose of the incision, whether in the abscess or cellulitis stage, is to evacuate and drain pus and bacteria accumulated in the underlying and surrounding tissues. Drainage of the cavity formed by the abscess significantly decreases the polybacterial load and necrotic debris found therein. The fact of decompressing the tissues and generating the evacuation results in reducing the hydrostatic pressure in the affected area, which allows the local blood supply and significantly increases the supply of immune defenses and antibiotics to the infected area. [11]

The incision of cellulitis functions to prevent the spread of bacterial infection to deeper anatomical planes. The incision procedure should include the placement of a drain to prevent premature closure of the previously performed dissection in order to prevent recurrence of the abscessed cavity and to allow for continued drainage. It is essential to keep in mind that the main surgical objective is to achieve adequate and sufficient drainage. [11]

The technique for intraoral incision will be based directly in a plane above the area of maximum fluctuation and inflammation. It is important to avoid the option of making the incision through a frenulum or through the path of the mentonian or inferior alveolar nerve.

When extraoral surgery is performed, a more complex set of criteria must be executed in order to correctly select the incision site. Once determined, pain control methods such as analgesics and anti-inflammatory drugs should be applied. [11]

The method of first choice is regional nerve block anesthesia, provided that infiltration of the anesthetic can be achieved in an area away from the infected area. Optionally, local infiltration of the anesthetic solution can be performed in and around the area to be surgically treated. It is essential that once the surgeon has used an anesthetic needle in an infected area, it is not reused in another non-infected area. [11]

Before carrying out the surgical procedure of the abscess or cellulitis, a sample should be obtained for subsequent culture by the microbiology department and have it ready and close to the surgical field.

Once the surgical area to be treated has been infiltrated and anesthetized, the superficial mucosa or superficial skin is disinfected with a solution, such as povidone iodine, and then dried with a sterile gauze with raytex identifier. [11]

To obtain the sample for the biological culture, a large gauge needle can be used, usually 18 gauge. It is suggested to use a small content syringe, generally of 3 ml or 5ml. Another option is the Stuart type swabs.

Subsequently, the needle is incised into the abscess or cellulitis and 1 to 2 ml of pus or fluid is aspirated. The sample may contain only fluid and blood instead of pus, commonly the sample provides sufficient quantity of bacteria for a good quality culture and study. [11]

The sample is placed in sterile tubes containing a swab and a specific transport medium and, under the appropriate conditions for bacteria, is inoculated directly into special containers for aerobic and anaerobic microorganisms to obtain samples.

All swab tubes and vials for the production and collection of samples have a limited shelf life, so it is necessary to check their expiration date before use. Care should be taken to keep the culture tubes in a continuous vertical position to avoid leakage of the carbon dioxide needed to preserve the anaerobic atmosphere inside the tube. [11]

Once the sample for culture has been obtained, with a scalpel blade, usually n.15, an incision is made between the mucosa and the submucosa until reaching the abscessed and infected cavity. The incision should be short, generally no longer than 1 cm. After the incision has been made, a closed curved hemostat (Kelly) is inserted through the incision until the target, the abscess cavity, is reached. In the next step, the hemostat is opened in different directions in order to break the small barriers, loculations or cavities of pus formed that could not be opened by the initial incision. The presence of pus or tissue fluid that drains during this time should be aspirated with the surgical aspirator and not allowed to drain freely into the patient's oral cavity. [11]

Once all areas of the abscess or cellulitis cavity have been dissected and all pus has been removed from them, a small drainage tube is placed to maintain the opening in the surgical incision. The most commonly used drainage for intraoral or extraoral abscesses is a sterile 0.6 cm long Pen rose drain.

An alternative that can often be used when such supplies are not available is a small sterile strip of rubber dam or latex surgical glove material. When selecting this surgical material, consideration should be given to the sensitivity that latex may have on the patient. [11]

A piece of drainage is made with the necessary length to reach the depth of the abscess or cellulitis cavity and is inserted in this surgical bed with the help of a hemostat mentioned above. Subsequently, the drainage is sutured on one edge of the previously made incision, with a non-absorbable stitch. The suture must be performed on viable and non-infected tissue, to avoid the loss of the drainage which could tear if it is positioned in devitalized and non-viable tissue. [11]

The drain should remain in the bed until there is no more material coming out of the abscess, usually this happens in the best conditions between 2 and 5 days. Removal and removal of the drain is accomplished by cutting the stitch and sliding the drain out of the surgical wound. [11]

Rationale 5: Pharmacological treatment of the patient.

The medical care required for the patient diagnosed with severe odontogenic infection is based mainly on 3 pillars: hydration, nutrition and control of hyperthermia. The maintenance and reestablishment of electrolyte balance in the patient as well as the control of systemic diseases represent a fundamental and crucial part of the medical care and support necessary for the patient. [14]

At temperatures above 38°, hyperthermia may be impaired as metabolic and cardiovascular demands increase beyond the patient's physiological reserve capacity. The patient's energy reserves can and tends to be rapidly depleted, as fluid loss increases dramatically. [14]

The daily loss of sensible fluids is constituted mainly by sweating which generates a loss of quantity of approximately 250 ml per degree of fever. The insensible fluid loss, which is constituted mainly by evaporation from the lungs and skin, increases from 50 to 75 ml per degree of fever per day. [14]

Hyperthermia results in an increase in metabolic demand of 5 to 8% per degree of fever per day. Therefore, it is necessary to supplement and replace the oral intake of the operated and hyperemic patient, probably the oral route can be intervened and significantly compromised by the local effects of acute infection and surgery, it may benefit from the use of supplementary feeding or even enteral nutrition through a nasogastric feeding tube. [14]

Rationale 6: Prescribing the appropriate antibiotic.

Odontogenic infections take their etiology from a known and predicted group of certain bacteria; the degree of antibiotic sensitivity against this type of microorganisms is well known and constant.

A daily therapeutic procedure consists of using antibiotics empirically, which involves administering the antibiotic with the objective of assuming that the appropriate drug is being administered according to the type of infection, the area of infection and the microorganisms usually present in it. [11]

Commonly the drug of choice is penicillin. The alternatives to be used in patients allergic to penicillin are clindamycin, cephalosporins and some macrolides. On the other hand, metronidazole has a useful indication only against bacteria of anaerobic origin and its use should be reserved for situations in which the exclusive presence of anaerobes is precisely identified or it should be administered in combination with another antibiotic, such as penicillin, to exert a synergistic effect and present activity against aerobic bacteria, or when other antibiotics are contraindicated. [11]

Laboratory studies showing antibiogram and sensitivity to certain antibiotics are informative, but cannot explain the effects of surgical treatment, bacterial interactions and immune response on the clinical situation. [11]

The results of several systematic reviews allow us to reach the following conclusion:

- Laboratory studies describing the antibiotic sensitivity of bacterial isolates from orofacial odontogenic infections indicate that newer, broader-spectrum antibiotics are more effective in vitro than older, narrower-spectrum antibiotics. [23]

See table n.7 Antibiotics of choice for empirical therapy. [23]

Antibiotics of choice for empiric therapy.	
Severity/Hypersensitivity	Antibiotics of choice
Ambulatory	Amoxicillin Clindamycin Azithromycin
Penicillin hypersensitivity	Clindamycin Azithromycin Azithromycin Metronidazole Moxifloxacin
Hospitalization	Ampicillin + sulbactam Clindamycin Penicillin + metronidazole Ceftriaxone
Penicillin hypersensitivity	Clindamycin Moxifloxacin Vancomycin + metronidazole

- Therefore, it seems reasonable to conclude that when combined with appropriate surgery, including incision, drainage and removal of the septic focus or even root canal treatment, the prognosis and use of these will benefit and may be favorable. [23]

- B-lactam antibiotics have an excellent safety profile, provided that an allergic reaction has been ruled out by a thorough review of the clinical history. [23]

- In a prospective case series of severe odontogenic infections requiring hospitalization, Flynn and colleagues found an intravenous penicillin G therapeutic failure rate of 21% in severe cases of odontogenic infection in hospitalized patients, and penicillin-resistant strains of infection were isolated from 54% of cases. [23]

- Al-Nawas and colleagues found an increased rate of penicillin resistance in inpatient and outpatient odontogenic infections. These findings indicate that it may be prudent to use a combination of a b-lactamase inhibitor drug, such as ampicillin/sulbactam, first-line in severe odontogenic infections requiring hospitalization. [23]

- In the case of penicillin allergy, clindamycin replaces b-lactam antibiotics as the drug of choice for safety reasons and because it has a broad spectrum. Antibiotic-associated colitis (AAC) caused by *Clostridium difficile* overgrowth is a concern in the therapeutic overuse of clindamycin. However, the demographics of odontogenic infections do not match those most commonly associated with AAC, which include prolonged hospitalization, abdominal surgery, advanced age, female gender, and multiple comorbidities. [23]

- Among the macrolide antibiotics, azithromycin has a lower drug-drug interaction rate than clarithromycin and erythromycin. Because azithromycin is metabolized by a different pathway than other macrolides, it bypasses CYP3A4, the hepatic microsomal enzyme most frequently associated with drug-drug interactions. [23]

- Metronidazole has been shown to be as effective as penicillin when used alone in outpatient odontogenic infections, when combined with appropriate surgery, even though it kills only anaerobic bacteria. In hospital infections, the combination of metronidazole with penicillin should be effective against almost all odontogenic pathogens. Recall that this combination crosses the blood-brain barrier. [23]

- Moxifloxacin is a fourth generation fluoroquinolone that is effective against Streptococci and oral anaerobes. Another advantage of this drug is its excellent absorption and bone penetration when administered orally. It should be avoided in pregnant women and children due to its toxicity to growing cartilage. [23]

- It has also been demonstrated in laboratory studies that cephalosporins are effective in odontogenic infections. [23]

- Among the antibiotics commonly used for odontogenic infections, it appears that no single antibiotic is clearly superior to all others. Therefore, antibiotics can be chosen according to cost and safety, with individualized consideration of the patient's medical history. Surgical treatment, consisting of incision and drainage and removal of the odontogenic cause by extraction, endodontic therapy or other means, is of paramount importance. [23]

Rationale 7: : Administer antibiotics appropriately.

Ideally, plasma concentrations should be high enough to inhibit the growth of bacteria that are sensitive to the antibiotic but without reaching levels that cause toxicity in the patient. [11]

Usually, the maximum plasma concentration of the drug should be at least four to five times higher than the minimum inhibitory concentration against the microorganisms and bacteria involved in the infection. [11]

Rationale 8: Frequently evaluate the patient.

In severe head and neck infections, close and continuous clinical follow-up from initial therapy is warranted because:

(1) Infections of odontogenic origin can and tend to progress to deeper anatomic spaces even after prior and complete drainage of all spaces affected by cellulitis or abscesses.

(2) There is a possibility that a failure of the host response to odontogenic infection may occur and be present, taking into account the context of the comorbidities that exist and compromise the patient's immune system.

(3) The incidence of antibiotic-resistant bacteria in head and neck infections is currently increasing. [11]

Criteria to be considered for hospital discharge include certain measures indicating a decrease in odontogenic infection, a stable and out-of-hazard airway, and recovery of full autonomic function by the patient. [11]

When an anatomical cause or septic focus of the clinical deterioration has not been identified, medical attention should be directed to a microbiological, systemic or immunological problem. In this case, an interconsultation with other specialists can be extremely useful. [11]

See table n.8 where the criteria to be considered for hospital discharge in a deep neck abscess are listed. [11]

<table>
<tr><td>Criteria for hospital discharge in deep neck abscess.</td></tr>
<tr><td>○ Complete and safe patient extubation</td></tr>
<tr><td>○ Temperature less than 37.8 for 24 hours</td></tr>
<tr><td>○ Permeable oral route</td></tr>
<tr><td>○ Removal of drains</td></tr>
<tr><td>○ Decrease in inflammation</td></tr>
<tr><td>○ Minimal or no drainage</td></tr>
<tr><td>○ Adequate systemic control</td></tr>
<tr><td>○ Ambulation</td></tr>
</table>

See table n. 9 Possible causes of treatment failure in patients with deep neck abscess. [15]

<table>
<tr><td>Possible causes of treatment failure.</td></tr>
</table>

CAUSER	EXAMPLE
Inadequate surgery	Inadequate surgical drainage.
Undiagnosed osteomyelitis	Recurrent soft tissue infection in contiguous anatomical spaces.
Immunosuppression	Poor metabolic control, HIV, leukemia, chemotherapy/radiation therapy, etc.
Presence of foreign body	Presence of implants.
Tumor	Squamous cell carcinoma.
Anatomical obstruction to drainage	Sialolithiasis, sinusitis.
Inadequate antibiotic selection	Incorrect choice of empirical antibiotic. Lack of follow-up and administration by the patient. Drug interactions. Incorrect dosage prescription. Error in the diagnosis of the culture.

Over-infection	Post-antibiotic candidiasis.
Re-infection	Actinomyces relapse.

1) PROTOCOL OF CARE FOR PATIENTS WITH DEEP NECK ABSCESS OF DENTAL ORIGIN AT THE XOCO GENERAL HOSPITAL.

1. Admit patient to the ER.

    a. The patient's medical history is taken and informed consent is obtained.
    b. The patient is cannulated through a peripheral permeable line (the need for a central venous catheter is assessed by the Emergency Department).
    c. Prescription of double antibiotic therapy empirically.
    d. The airway is assessed (the need for orotracheal intubation for airway protection is determined if necessary by the Emergency Department).
    e. A diagnosis was made by the Emergency Department and a referral was made to the Maxillofacial and Reconstructive Plastic Surgery Department (MRCPD).

2. Elaboration of a note of evaluation and admission by the CPR and Maxillofacial service.

    a. Laboratories are requested: blood cytometry, blood chemistry, prothrombin time (PT), thromboplastin time (PTT), international normalized ratio (INR), serum electrolytes.
    b. Imaging studies were requested: simple computed tomography of the facial mass, with extension to the neck and thorax.
    c. The extension and dissemination of the infectious process to the involved anatomical aponeurotic spaces is established, determining the degree of severity.
    d. The request and consent for surgical intervention is given to the patient.

e. Request for surgical time in the operating room for incision procedure, drainage and removal of septic focus.

3. If the patient is older than 40 years old, he/she is referred to the Internal Medicine Department for pre-surgical systemic evaluation.

4. The anesthesiology department is consulted for preoperative evaluation of the patient.

   a. Assessment of health status based on laboratory results.
   b. Airway assessment.
   b.1 If the Anesthesiology service determines that the airway is difficult, the patient is referred to the Endoscopy service for intubation with nasofibroendoscopy.

   c. Balanced general anesthesia/sedation.
   d. The patient is intubated according to the Anesthesiology treatment plan (nasotracheal, orotracheal).

5. Consultation with the General Surgery Service (when it is determined that the airway must be protected to perform the surgical procedure of tracheostomy).

See Annex 1: Definition and indications for tracheostomy and tracheotomy.
See Annex 2: Tracheotomy surgical technique.

6. Admission to operating room for contaminated procedures.

7. Verification of safe surgery with nursing, medical and surgical staff.

8. Surgical techniques of asepsis and antisepsis.

9. Infiltration under local regional anesthesia.

10. Extraction of septic focus (extraction of the involved tooth).

11. Incision according to the principles of authors Topazian, Laskin and Petterson.

12. Blunt dissection.

Incision and dissection for drainage of deep neck abscess.

a. Incision with a scalpel, preferably with a number 15 blade.

b. Incision in healthy tissue, it should not be performed in the most fluctuant area of the abscess or cellulitis (in order to obtain an adequate healing and avoid sloughing).

c. Incision in an area where drainage is facilitated by gravity.

d. Incision in aesthetic areas (marginal mandibular border, at the level of the formation of a natural skin fold whenever convenient).

e. Blunt dissection, with closed kelly scissors, through the deep tissues and exploring in all possible directions, with the objective of accessing compartmentalized areas occupied by pus, extending the dissection to the levels of the tooth apices of the teeth involved; if necessary, the debridement of several anatomical spaces can be performed by communicating spaces through the incision (using digito-dissection). [24]

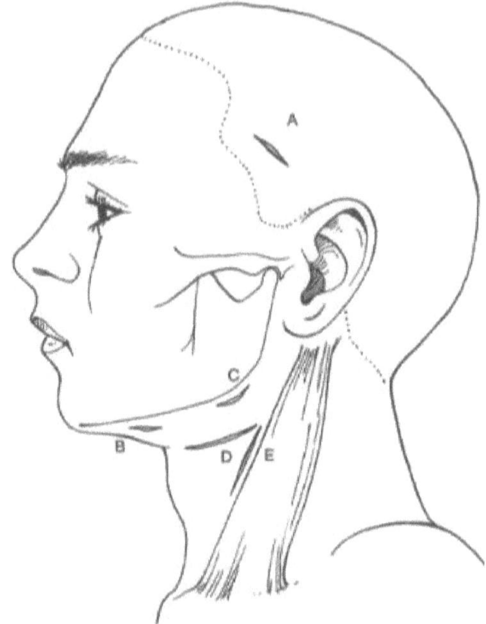

Fig. n. 3 Proposed lines for extraoral incision in deep neck abscess.
A: Temporal superficial or deep.
B: Submental or submandibular.
C: Submandibular, Submaseteric or Pterygomandibular.
D: Lateral pharyngeal or superior retropharyngeal.
E: Retropharyngeal or carotid vein region. [25]

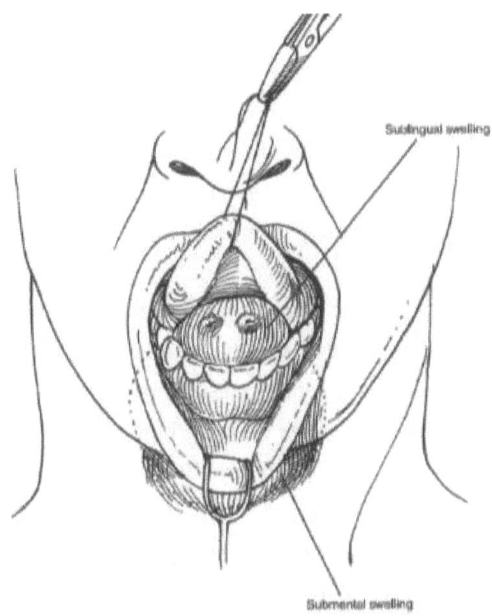

Fig. n. 4 Sublingual and submental space occupied by an odontogenic infection. [25]

13. Culture was taken and transferred to the Microbiology Department of the General Hospital of Xoco.

Crop intake and crop transfer.

Oral and maxillofacial infections represent a unique problem due to the abundance and variety of organisms present in this region as well as the changing nature observed in recent years. Saliva contains approximately one hundred million anaerobic species and ten million aerobic species and facultative anaerobic organisms. This creates a great risk of contamination and over-infection. Different categories of microorganisms are responsible for the etiology of infections of dental origin among them are distinguished: aerobes, anaerobes, acid-fast bacteria, fungi, viruses, spirochetes, etc.

In general, a clinical diagnosis of an infection must be confirmed with laboratory studies. Cultures to detect the type of microorganisms present in an infectious process require at least 24 hours to study their development and growth and up to 48 hours for the development of *fungi, mycoplasma or chlamydia.*

Specimen collection and transport.

Proper culture collection of the specimen to be studied means optimal transport and culture collection. An inadequate maneuver in culture handling can lead to an erroneous diagnosis and treatment, having to repeat the sample collection days later.

Microorganisms representative of the area of active infection should be collected in an adequate and sufficient manner. Inadequate containers or means of transport may cause contamination of the sample or the person taking it, as well as loss of viability of the microorganisms.

Aseptic preparation techniques are important in lesions exposed or contiguous to the oropharyngeal or cutaneous area in order to minimize the introduction, contamination and colonization of microorganisms in the study culture. Irrigation with saline or sterile water is essential. Antiseptics should not be used because they can cause the death of bacteria before they can be transported and studied in the culture.

Lesions with accumulation of detritus or necrotic tissue can be previously cleaned with soap that has a minimal antibacterial effect and then irrigated.

Stuart's, Amie's or Cary Blair are means of transport that currently exist for further study in a culture medium.

A maximum lapse of 2 hours is allowed between taking the culture and the microbiological examination of the specimen. This results in progressive loss of viability, disproportionate growth, alteration in the morphology of the microorganisms, etc. Refrigeration should be used only when there is no other alternative; many organisms die due to inadequate handling such as inadequate temperature and loss of the protocol for their study. [27]

Photographs taken at the Microbiology Department of the Xoco General Hospital.

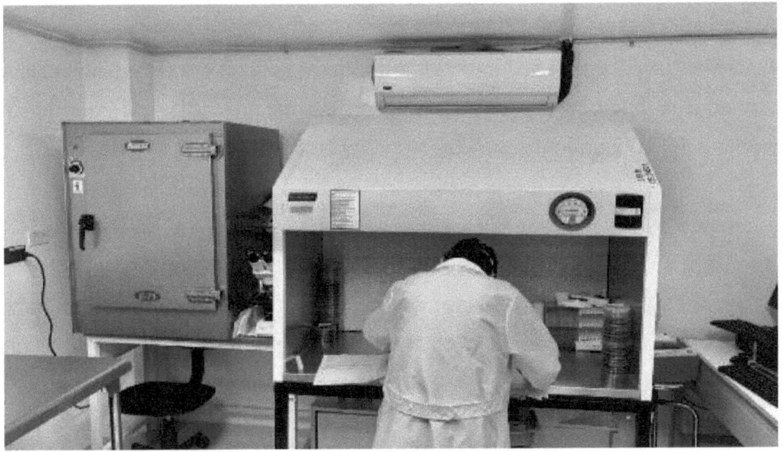

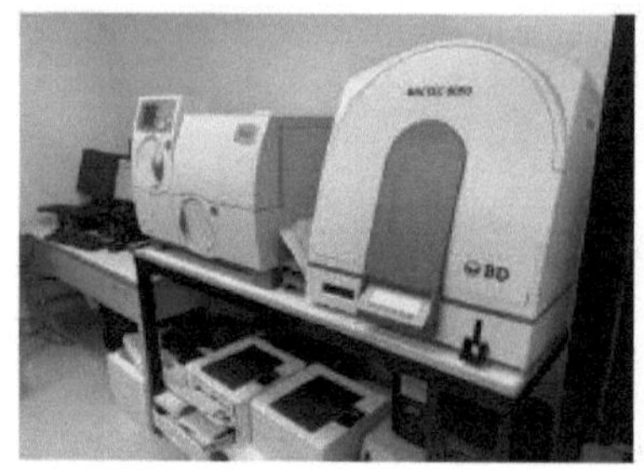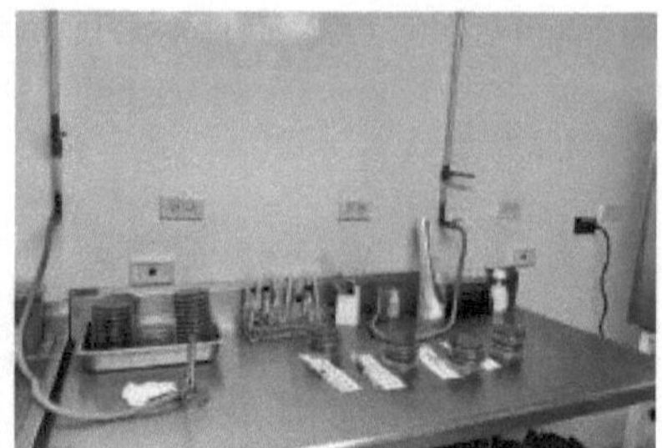

14. Drainage.

15. Placement of Pen rose drain.

Drainage and lavage in deep neck abscess. Definition, indications and placement of Pen Rose.

All anatomical spaces involved in a process of cellulitis or abscess caused by an odontogenic infection should be drained as soon as possible. Drainage at the cellulitis stage has been shown to prevent the spread of the infection to contiguous and deep anatomical spaces of the neck, also favoring the taking of cultures at this stage for the early detection of the microorganisms present in it.

Debridement and irrigation of infected anatomical spaces are aimed at reducing the amount of bacteria present, as well as the elimination of necrotic tissue, preventing the subsequent colonization of antibiotic-resistant bacteria.

The purpose of the drainage is to achieve the expulsion of the hematic-purulent content in favor of gravity through the incision and placement of the Pen rose drain, as well as to favor the debridement of the infected area through continuous irrigation with a thirds solution (iodine, hydrogen peroxide, physiological solution). Drains (Pen rose, Jackson-Pratt, latex) are usually removed from the surgical wound within 2 to 7 days. [25]

Pen rose drainage

Drains are materials designed to channel unwanted fluids and/or air from tissues or body cavities.

There are three main indications for placement:

1) To facilitate the elimination of dead space.
2) Evacuate existing accumulations of fluids and/or gases.
3) Prevent early formation of fluid accumulations.

They are soft, malleable, radiopaque, readily available, economical, biocompatible, and are resistant to high temperatures allowing them to be sterilized. Pen rose drains are available in lengths of 30 to 45 cm (12-18 inches) and in widths of 6 to 25 mm. Although tubular, most drainage occurs extraluminally and is driven by gravity and capillary action. The amount of drainage is proportional to the surface area of the Pen rose drainage.

This drain is useful for thick viscous fluids, which often clog the lumen of smaller drains. Pen rose drains should not be perforated, as this reduces the surface area, decreasing drainage efficiency.

Perforations also weaken the drain and allow adhesions to develop between the drain and the soft tissues, which can result in the drain rupturing when traction is applied to remove it.

Pen rose drains can be used successfully in wounds that cannot be completely debrided and in the presence of debris and foreign material, massively contaminated tissue, and fluid-filled dead spaces.

The drain must be placed and maintained under aseptic conditions. The implantation site should be aseptically prepared and, if necessary, infiltrated with local anesthesia. The most direct and shortest route for fluid evacuation should be selected.

Passive drainage is introduced into the wound from the inside out, minimizing skin contamination. The drain is placed deep into the tissue in need of drainage and anchored to the skin to prevent dislodgement. A single stitch is placed. The suture is placed from the skin to the wound, through the drain.

The drainage end must be long enough to evacuate fluids and to prevent their retraction into the wound when the patient moves. [26]

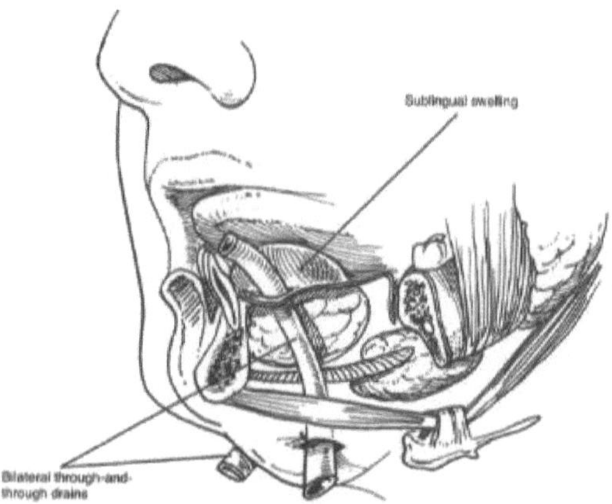

Fig. n.5 Pen rose drain placement communicating the submental space with the sublingual space.

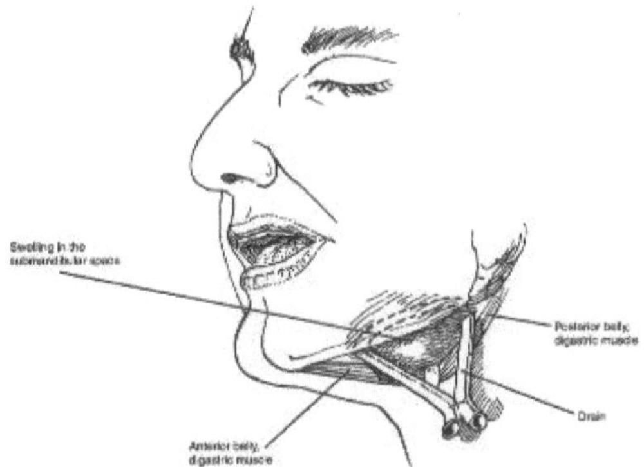

Fig. n. 6 Placement of Pen rose type drainage communicating the submental space with the sublingual space.

16. Washing and surgical transoperative cleaning with thirds solution (Iodopovidone, hydrogen peroxide, physiological solution).

17. Surgical wound is covered with cervical bandage.

18. Transfer of the patient to the recovery area.

19. Elaboration of operative and postoperative notes.

20. Elaboration of postoperative indications. (Admission of the patient to the Intensive Care Unit in case it has been decided by the surgical doctors).

21. Physical and clinical assessment based on laboratory results, to determine the evolution of the intervened patient.

Determination of the evolution of the intervened patient.

In ambulatory infections that have been treated by extraction of the septic focus. Example: one tooth or several teeth, incision and intraoral drainage, the optimal follow-up appointment is usually 2 days postoperatively for the following reasons:

1. Drainage has usually ceased and drainage may be discontinued at this time.

2. There is usually a noticeable improvement or deterioration in signs and symptoms that allow the following treatment decisions to be made.

For odontogenic infections involving deep anatomic spaces that are severe enough for hospitalization, daily clinical evaluation and wound healing is required. By 2 to 3 days postoperatively, clinical signs of improvement should be evident, such as decreased swelling, decreased wound drainage, decreased white blood cell count, decreased discomfort and pain as well as decreased airway inflammation, so extubation can be considered. Preliminary culture results should also be available at this time, which may provide some guidance on the assertiveness of empiric antibiotic therapy.

If the above signs of clinical improvement are not evident, then it should be necessary to begin an investigation for possible treatment failure.

One of the most efficient methods is postoperative CT reevaluation. A postoperative CT scan may show continued airway inflammation that may prevent extubation or further spread of infection to previously undrained anatomic spaces, or it may also confirm adequate surgical drainage of all affected anatomic spaces by visualization of radiopaque drains in all affected anatomic spaces. [6]

According to an article published in the Journal of Cranio-Maxillo-Facial Surgery in 2018 named: the role of c-reactive protein and white blood cell count for prediction in hospital stay and severity of odontogenic abscess; levels of C-Reactive Protein and leukocyte counts quantified preemptively may be predictive factors for hospital stay in long-term hospitalized patients.[21]

6. Clinical case report.

Male patient, 38 years old, with the initials J.A.N.S. Hereditary and non-pathological family history with no relevance to the current condition. Personal pathological history: Obesity grade III, denies chronic degenerative diseases. The current condition began 10 days before, referring to a failed attempt to extract the lower left third molar with a physician. Subsequently, she evolves with an increase of volume in the left submandibular region, referring dental pain, difficulty in speaking and swallowing of 1 day of evolution, treated with clindamycin and dexamethasone by the same physician, without resolution. On July 19, 2021, she went to the emergency department of the General Hospital of Xoco where she was diagnosed with deep neck abscess in the left submandibular, submental, bilateral sublingual and left parapharyngeal anatomical area.

On admission the patient presented general malaise, tachypnea, body hyperthermia of 38°, limited mouth opening, dyspnea, odynophagia, dysphagia, dysphonia, stridor and hot potato voice. In the sublingual, left submandibular and submental areas there was an erythematous increase in volume with fluctuating consistency and hyperemic on palpation. Intraorally there is an elevated floor of the mouth, difficulty to mobilize the tongue, and deviation of the uvula to the right side. *See image 1.*

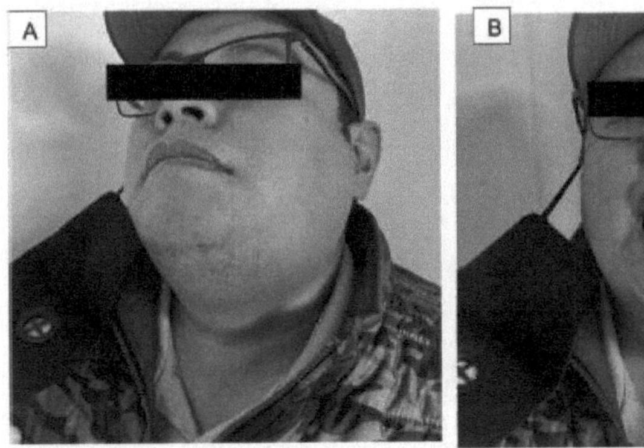

Image n.1 **Extraoral photographs of patient with deep neck abscess.**

A) Lateral view: **Increased volume is observed in sublingual, submandibular and submental region as well as peripheral erythematous areas.**

B) Frontal view: **Limitation in oral opening is observed when the patient is asked to perform maximum mouth opening.**

Care protocol is initiated for deep neck abscess:

A.   A peripheral permeable line was cannulated with physiological solution at 0.9% 1000cc for 24 hours, empirical antibiotic therapy was started with a double scheme with ceftriaxone 1 g IV every 12 hours and clindamycin 600 mg IV every 8 hours. For analgesia, paracetamol 1 g IV every 8 hours and ketorolac 30 mg IV every 8 hours are used. For gastric protection, omeprazole 40 mg IV every 24 hours is indicated.

B.   Results of laboratory studies were obtained: leukocytes: 22,000 cells x mm3 , hemoglobin 19.0 gr/dl, hematocrit 55.5 % glucose 83 mg/dl, creatinine 0.7 mg/dl, platelets 303,000 per microliter, PT 13.9 sec. PTT 26.0 sec. INR 1.15.

C.   A simple computed tomography (CT) scan of the facial mass with extension to the mediastinum was performed, showing isodense areas to soft tissues with displacement of the airway to the right, hypodense area to collection in the left parapharyngeal space, extending to the left submandibular, bilateral sublingual and submental areas (*fig. 3-7)*.

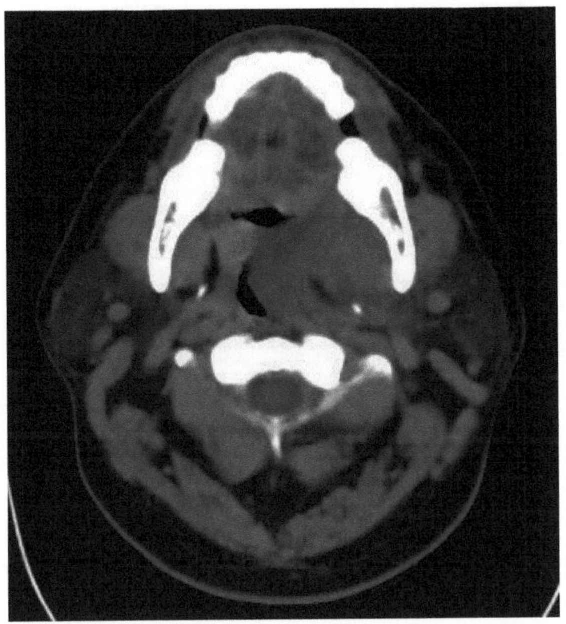

Fig. n. 3 CT of simple facial mass in axial section in window for soft tissues at the level of the mandibular angle where an isodense zone to soft tissues with displacement of airway to the right, hypodense zone to collection in left parapharyngeal space, extending to left submandibular, submental and bilateral sublingual zones can be seen.

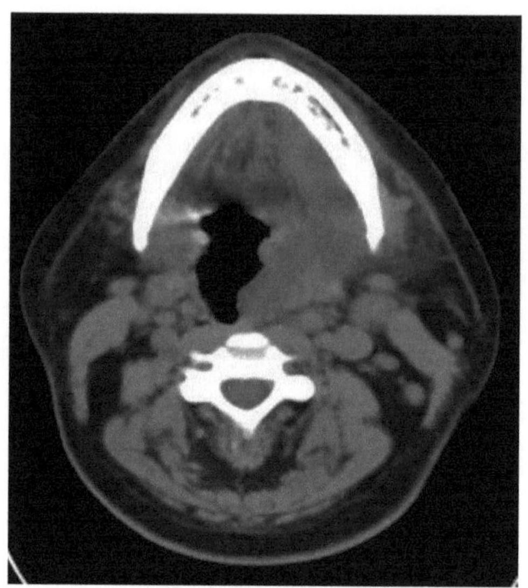

Fig. n. 4 CT of simple facial mass in axial section in window for soft tissues at the level of the mandibular body where an isodense zone to soft tissues with displacement of the airway to the right, hypodense zone to collection in the left submandibular space, extending towards the bilateral sublingual space can be seen.

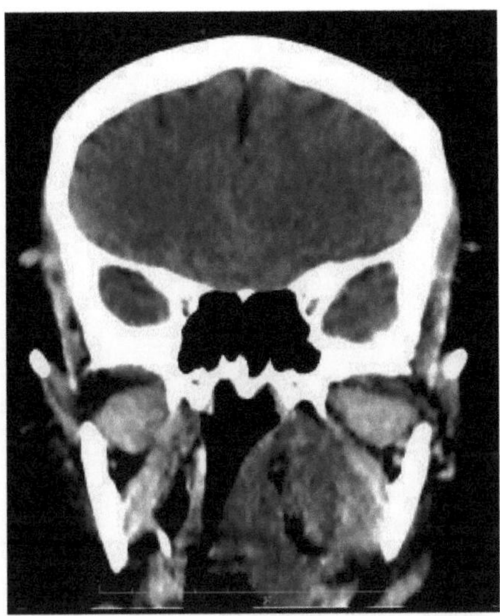

Fig. n. 5 CT of simple facial mass in coronal section at the level of the mandibular branches in soft tissue window where you can see isodense area to soft tissues in the left parapharyngeal region also presenting hypodense areas compatible with gas.

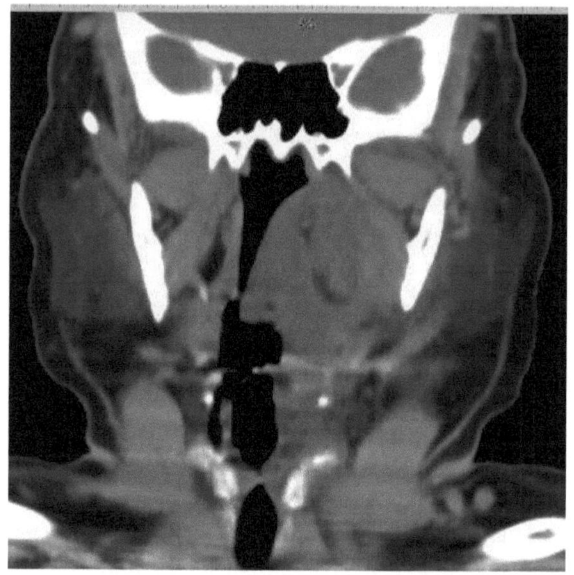

Fig. n. 6 CT of simple facial mass in coronal section at the level of the mandibular branches in soft tissues sale where the deviation towards the right side of the upper airway can be seen.

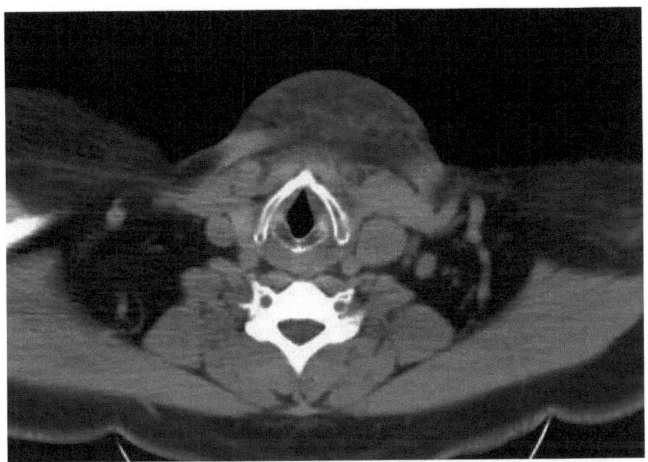

Fig. n. 7 CT of simple facial mass with extension to mediastinum in axial section at the level of the epiglottis, in which airway patency is observed, with absence of mediastinitis data.

D. The patient is admitted to the operating room together with the Anesthesiology, General Surgery and Maxillofacial and Reconstructive Plastic Surgery teams.

E. Under balanced general anesthesia and previous orotracheal intubation, a tracheostomy procedure was started by the General Surgery service physicians to protect the airway and prevent airway collapse. Surgical time is continued for incision and abscess drainage by the Plastic Reconstructive and Maxillofacial Surgery service *(fig. n.8)*.

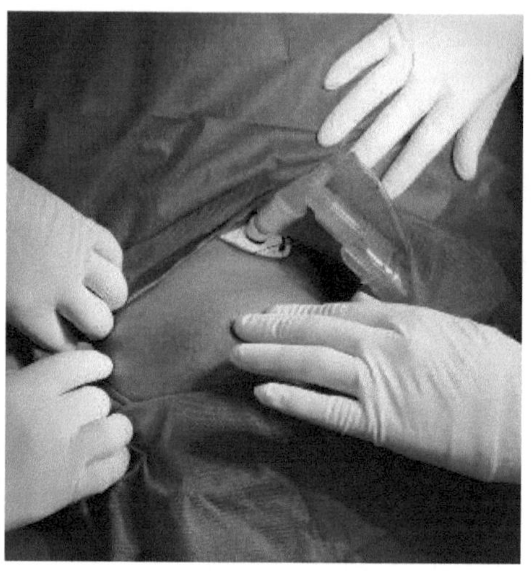

Fig. n.8 Tracheostomy connected to artificial respirator.

F. The septic focus (lower left third molar) was removed. Two incisions were made in the left submandibular and submental areas *(fig.9-10)*. Fasciotomies are performed with kelly forceps decompressing, communicating and draining the bilateral sublingual and left submandibular anatomical areas *(fig.11)* the latter is communicated with the lateral parapharyngeal space by means of digit dissection *(fig.12)*, obtaining an evacuation of frank purulent content of yellowish fetid color of approximately 35 cc. *(fig.12) A* culture is taken with antibiogram of the surgical bed *(fig.13)*. Subsequent irrigation and surgical cleaning.

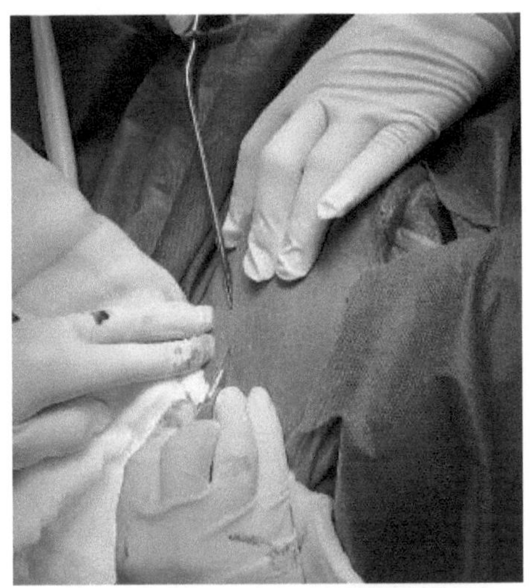

Fig. n. 9 Submandibular incision.

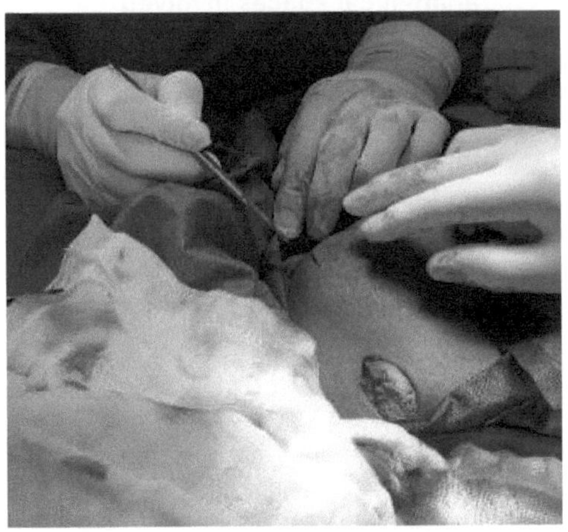

Fig. n. 10 Submental incision.

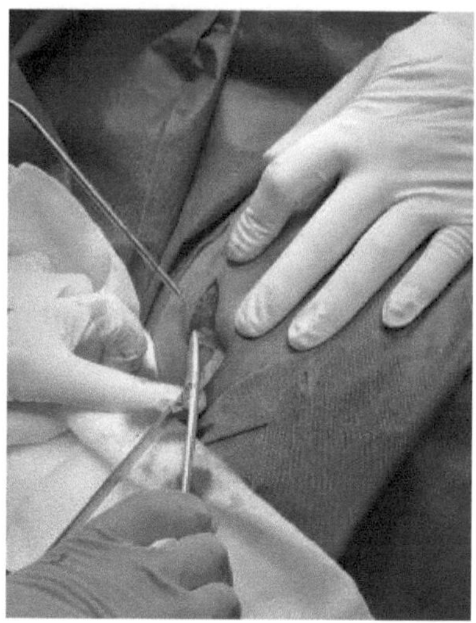

Fig. n. 11 Dissection by planes with Kelly forceps communicating anatomical spaces involved.

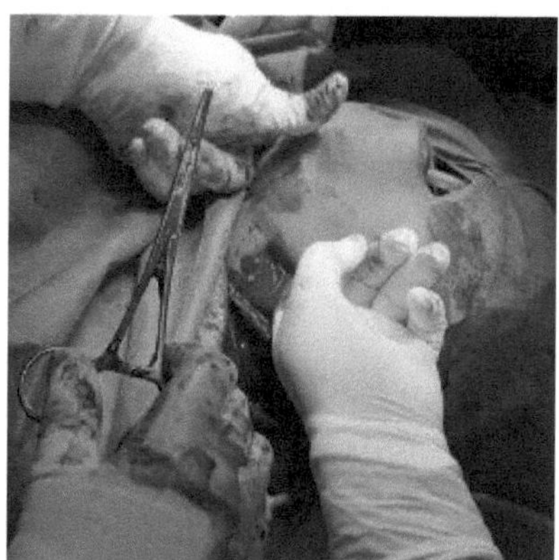

Fig. n. 12 Dissection digit where submandibular spaces communicate with the left parapharyngeal space, also showing evacuation of purulent hematic content of the abscess.

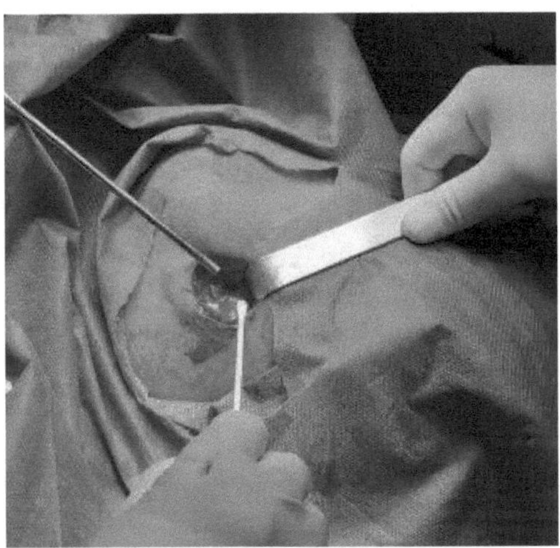

Fig. n. 13 Culture and antibiogram of the surgical site.

Two Penrose drainage tubes are placed to communicate the submental area with the left submandibular area, sutured with a simple silk stitch at both ends of the healthy skin tissue surrounding the operated area *(fig.14)*. Finally, a cervical bandage is applied to protect and cover the drains.

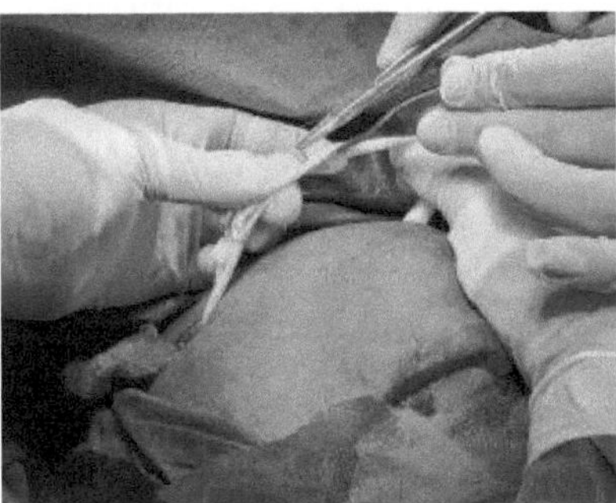

Fig. n. 14 Placement of Pen Rose drains communicating submandibular and submental area.

G. The patient is admitted to the intensive care and therapy unit (ICU) for close monitoring where it is decided to place a nasogastric tube for nutrition and feeding (*fig. 15*).

As per protocol, surgical wounds are healed with a thirds solution composed of iodine, hydrogen peroxide and physiological solution every 8 hours by the CPR and Maxillofacial service.

The Internal Medicine Department was consulted because the patient's blood pressure was higher than normal during the anesthetic event, and he was diagnosed with arterial hypertension and was treated with amlodipine 5 mg every 12 hours and captopril 25 mg every 12 hours.

The results of the culture showed *Staphylococcus hominis, so it was* decided to change the antibiotic to Imipenem 1g IV every 8 hours for 7 days because the bacteria showed sensitivity in the antibiogram.

On the third day of stay in the ICU, it was decided to make progression and withdraw mechanical ventilatory support.

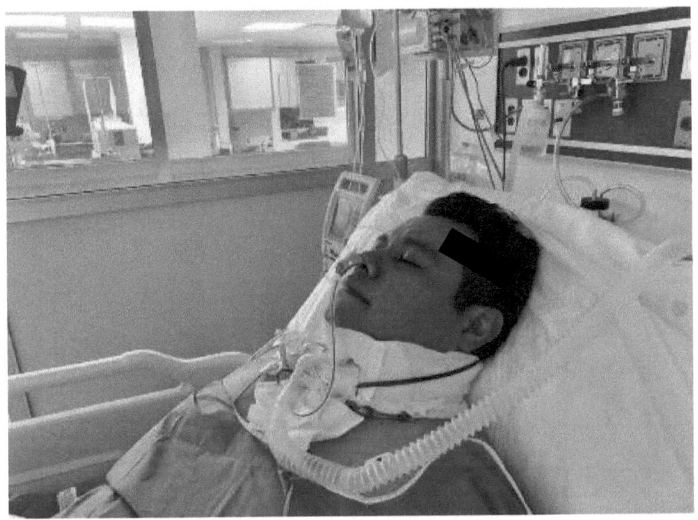

Fig. n. 15 Patient in the ICU after surgery.

H. Eleven days after admission, the patient was found with a Glasgow index of 15, without data of SIRS (Systemic Inflammatory Response Syndrome), hemodynamically integrated, it was decided to admit the patient to the floor of Maxillofacial and Reconstructive Plastic Surgery where tracheostomy progression was performed and the nasogastric tube was removed.

I. After 13 days of surgery and after completing the antibiotic regimen and noting evolution in his saturation (92% without supplemental oxygen), clinically presenting a correct confrontation of the cutaneous planes in the tracheostomy wound with edges free of active infection data, with a considerable decrease in the increase of volume in the area of the abscess previously drained, observing both surgical wounds free of infection data and free of any type of secretion.

With labs showing the following results: leukocytes 11,200 x mm3, hemoglobin 17.0 gr/dl, hematocrit 50.8%, glucose 72 mg/dl, creatinine 0.8 mg/dl, platelets 364,000 per microliter, PT 12.9 sec. TPT 31.8 sec. INR 1.17.

J. Hospital discharge was decided with antibiotic therapy and oral analgesia, surgical wound washings every 8 hours with neutral soap, strict oral hygiene, rinses with 0.12% chlorhexidine. With subsequent follow-up appointments in the outpatient clinic on the 3rd day of discharge from the General Hospital of Xoco.

Conclusions

One of the most controversial and discussed topics in the area of oral and maxillofacial surgery is whether or not to perform the extraction of the teeth involved at the time of the acute phase of the infection. The medical experience with the multiple patients admitted and operated with this diagnosis in the General Hospital of Xoco suggests that incision and drainage both in the cellulitic stage which is the moment of acute phase of the infection and in the abscess stage and tooth extraction are an important complement, which has resulted in a faster recovery of the host and a considerable decrease of the local bacterial load.

On the other hand, as mentioned in this work, the rapid increase as well as the decrease in the levels of c-reactive protein in acute inflammatory processes make it possible for this marker to be a predictable indicator of inflammation in the acute phase, representing a high sensitivity. In this work an obstacle was presented by the fact of not being able to quantify and report CRP levels at the time of hospital admission and discharge, because within the protocol of care of deep neck abscess in the General Hospital of Xoco this marker is not requested.

Let us remember that odontogenic infections take their origin from a known and predictable group of certain bacteria (either aerobic or anaerobic), the degree of sensitivity of these microorganisms to antibiotics is well known and constant. Therefore, the use of an empirical antibiotic regimen is intended to provide a rapid pharmacological therapy for the patient upon arrival at the hospital in order to reduce the acute infection and improve the patient's condition. Based on the fact that this antibiotic will be the appropriate one according to the infection and the anatomical area where the infection is occurring.

Early referral to the specialist is necessary for patients who have already been identified with some systemic involvement and in the course of developing a severe odontogenic infection, as these patients are part of the at-risk population and have a tendency to severity in a deep neck abscess.

Timely diagnosis and optimal treatment are key to reducing deaths associated with severe odontogenic infections.

The correct control of the patient's associated comorbidities may be a favorable prognostic reason in patients who develop deep neck abscess.

Initial empirical intravenous pharmacological impregnation, as well as continuous surgical drainage and lavage have been shown to be successful in the survival of patients with deep neck abscess at the General Hospital of Xoco. The multidisciplinary medical treatment of deep neck abscess represents an achievement in patient survival.

ANNEXES

ANNEX 1: Definition and indications for tracheostomy.

It is important to emphasize the diversification of the term tracheostomy from tracheotomy.

Tracheostomy is defined as a surgical technique that consists of creating an opening at the level of the cervical trachea, followed by the placement of a cannula that makes it impossible to close the incision just made and therefore allows the patient to continue breathing, in such a way that the passage of air through the upper airway is avoided, communicating the air from the external environment with the lower tracheal portion, bronchi and lungs.

The term tracheostomy is that surgical act that originates from the aforementioned opening of the trachea, through the placement of a cannula that aims to communicate the outside air with the lower airway, and therefore the generation of an artificial way of breathing. [3]

The dictionary of Medical Terms of the Royal Academy of Medicine defines tracheotomy as the incision of the trachea, while it defines tracheostomy as the opening of a hole in the trachea in order to allow breathing. [3]

The indications for tracheostomy can be manifested in different scenarios. The objective of tracheostomy is to provide a way for air to enter from the external environment into the lower airway, avoiding obstacles that may be present in the oral cavity, pharynx and larynx. [3]

Table 10 and 11 below lists two classifications indicating the indications for tracheostomy. [3]

Table n. 10 Indications to perform the tracheostomy procedure.

Mechanical obstruction	Obstruction by secretions, respiratory insufficiency or both	Respiratory failure on or after:	Retention of exudates with alveolar respiratory insufficiency
a) Tumors of the pharynx, larynx, trachea or esophagus.	a) Accumulation of exudates adherent or insufficient cough reflex.	a) Intoxication by drugs or poisons.	a) Systemic diseases central nervous system (stroke, encephalitis, poliomyelitis, tetanus).
b) Congenital malformations of the airway/upper gastrointestinal tract.	b) For interventions thoracic and abdominal.	b) Closed thoracic trauma with fracture of the thorax. ribs.	b) Eclampsia.
c) Trauma to the larynx, or trachea.	c) Bronchopneumonia.	c) Paralysis of the respiratory musculature.	c) Severe head trauma, cervical, thoracic.
d) Aspiration of foreign bodies.	d) Vomiting and aspiration of gastric contents.	d) Chronic diseases obstructive pulmonary diseases (emphysema, chronic bronchitis, bronchiectasis, asthma, atelectasis).	d) Postoperative neurosurgical coma.
e) Craniofacial trauma with soft tissue edema or fracture. of the jaw.	e) Burns of the face, neck and respiratory tree.		e) Gas or fat embolism.
f) Inflammations (edemas) of Laryngeal, trachea, tongue, pharynx Airway protection in deep neck abscesses.	f) Pre-coma states due to metabolic decontrol (diabetes, hepatic, renal).		

Table n. 11 Indications for tracheostomy according to AAOHNS.

Indications for tracheostomy according to the American Academy of Otolaryngology Head and Neck Surgery.	
1.	Prolonged orotracheal intubation or with the expectation of being prolonged.
2.	Inability of the patient to manage secretions.
3.	Facilitation of ventilatory support.
4.	Impossibility of intubation.
5.	Assistant in the management of or in head and neck surgery.
6.	Assistant in the management of severe head and neck trauma.

The procedure should be performed in an operating room, preferably under general anesthesia. If this situation is not possible, local anesthesia should be used; however, an anesthesiologist should always be present.

1. Prior to surgery, the patient should be placed in the dorsal decubitus position and the neck positioned in hyperextension, placing a roller under the shoulders, which aims to elevate the trachea.

2. Antisepsis techniques are performed on the skin tissue and local anesthesia is infiltrated in the area where the incision is to be made.

3. The laryngeal and tracheal anatomical structures are then located by manual palpation: the larynx is fixed with the 1st and 3rd fingers of the left hand and the thyroid cartilage together with its notch, the cricothyroid space, cricoid cartilage, and the first rings of the trachea are palpated with the index finger of the other hand.

4. As for the incision, generally, it can be performed by two techniques:

   a) Transverse incision or described as slightly arcuate with a smooth superior concavity, about 5 cm in length, as a reference one finger below the inferior border of the cricoid cartilage, or at the level of two fingers above the suprasternal recess. This type of incision is described as more esthetic but provides the surgeon with a narrow surgical field.

   b) Vertical incision, centered at midline level, performed in the safety zone which is limited below by the sternal fork; above by the cricoid cartilage and on both sides by the anterior borders of the sternocleidomastoid muscles. This type of incision, despite being described as a less esthetic incision, has the advantage of providing a wider surgical field.

5. The skin, the subcutaneous cellular tissue and the cutaneous muscle of the neck (platysma) are dissected.

6. The anterior layer of deep cervical aponeurosis is dissected and the prelaryngeal muscles (sternohyoid and sternothyroid) are separated. Sometimes it is necessary to ligate one or both anterior jugular veins at this level.

7. The albicans midline of the sternohyoid and sternothyroid muscles should be located and dissection should be performed at this level.

8. The posterior layer of the deep cervical aponeurosis is incised, where the isthmus of the thyroid gland appears, this can reach up to the 3rd or 4th ring of the trachea, it is usually sectioned and ligated with sutures to adequately expose the trachea technique described as transisthmic tracheotomy, sometimes it can be moved cranially (infra-isthmic tracheotomy) or caudally (supra-isthmic tracheotomy).

9. On both sides of the trachea runs the vasculonervous bundle of the neck composed of: the carotid artery, the internal jugular vein and the vagus nerve and immediately behind the trachea is the esophagus. Under normal conditions they are not usually damaged, but when there are tumorous, inflammatory or traumatic processes of the neck, extreme precautions must be taken.

10. The anterior wall of the trachea is infiltrated with local anesthesia to avoid inhibitory reflexes when accessing the trachea.

11.   The trachea is incised through a vertical incision in the child or horizontal in the adult, resecting a window of the tracheal cartilage or making a U-shaped flap, avoiding if possible to cut the endotracheal tube balloon, and leaving undamaged at least one tracheal ring below the cricoid cartilage, ideally it should be opened at the level of the 3rd tracheal ring. When tracheostomy is performed at a very high level (close to the cricoid cartilage), there is a risk of subglottic stenosis, which is difficult to treat. A tracheotomy at a very low level has the risk of massive hemorrhage due to brachiocephalic trunk injury.

12. The trachea is fixed to the skin with silk stitches on the upper and lower edge that include the skin, subcutaneous cellular tissue and tracheal wall.

13. When accessing the trachea, the orotracheal tube is deflated and slowly withdrawn, just above the incision without removing it.

14. The appropriately sized cannula is introduced with its blunt guide, after verifying the condition of the balloon.

15. Once in place, secretions or blood are aspirated with a flexible tube and the ventilation circuit is changed to the cannula.

16. Once adequate ventilation and oxygenation of the patient is confirmed, the retractors and endotracheal tube are removed. The cannula is usually number 7 or 8 in adults. In children, cannulae number 2 to 5 are usually used. The cannula balloon should be inflated when appropriate, according to the patient's pathology, and to the extent deemed necessary.

17. Finally, the hemostasis is thoroughly checked and the skin is sutured on each side with 1 or 2 silk stitches.

18. The bib and the specific straps to hold the tracheal cannula around the neck are placed and immediate post-operative care is performed. [3]

8. Bibliographical references.

1.Levy M. Intraperitoneal drainage. Am J Surg [Internet].
1984;147(3):309–14. Disponible en:
https://www.sciencedirect.com/science/article/pii/0002961084901569
1.

2.Robinson JO. Surgical drainage: an historical perspective. Br J Surg
[Internet]. 1986;73(6):422–6. Disponible en:
http://dx.doi.org/10.1002/bjs.1800730603

3. García AC. Manual de manejo de la traqueotomía para Sanitarios y
Pacientes. Algeciras: LiberLIBRO; 2014.

4. Drenajes abdominales: una breve reseña histórica. Irish medi.
2001;94(6):164–6.

5. Fating NS, Saikrishna D, Vijay Kumar GS, Shetty SK, Raghavendra
Rao M. Detection of bacterial flora in orofacial space infections and
their antibiotic sensitivity profile. J Maxillofac Oral Surg [Internet].
2014;13(4):525–32. Disponible en: http://dx.doi.org/10.1007/s12663-
013-0575-7

6. Peterson LJ. Contemporary management of deep infections of the
neck. J Oral Maxillofac Surg [Internet]. 1993;51(3):226–31. Disponible
en:
https://www.sciencedirect.com/science/article/pii/S0278239110801624

7. Parthiban S, Muthukumar R, Karthi M. Ludwig's Angina: A Rare
Case Report [Internet]. Vol. 2, Indian Journal of Multidisciplinary
Dentistry; Chennai volume. 2012. Disponible en:

https://www.proquest.com/openview/61d00b025338d589404e13fee3e
a2e33/1?pq-origsite=gscholar&cbl=1316336

8. Nicolaou KC, Rigol S. A brief history of antibiotics and select
advances in their synthesis. J Antibiot (Tokyo) [Internet]. 2018 [citado
el 25 de febrero de 2022];71(2):153–84. Disponible en:
https://www.nature.com/articles/ja201762

9. Thompson. SH. Anatomy Relevant to Head, Neck, and Orofacial
Infections. En: Head neck and Orofacial Infections. St. Louis Missouri:
Elsevier; 2016. p. 60–93.

10. Ferneini EM, Goldberg MH. Management of oral and maxillofacial
infections. J Oral Maxillofac Surg [Internet]. 2018 [citado el 25 de
febrero de 2022];76(3):469–73. Disponible en:
https://www.joms.org/article/S0278-2391(17)31452-0/fulltext

11. Flynn TR. Fundamentos del tratamiento y la prevención de las
infecciones odontogénicas. In: Cirugía Oral y Maxilofacial
Contemporánea. Barcelona, Spain: Elsevier Masson; 2014.

12. Dinulos JGH, Pace NC. Bacterial Infections. In: Eichenfield LF,
Frieden IJ, Esterly NB, editors. Neonatal Dermatology. Toronto, ON,
Canada: Elsevier; 2008. p. 173–91.

13. Karkos PD, Leong SC, Beer H, Apostolidou MT, Panarese A.
Challenging airways in deep neck space infections. Am J Otolaryngol
[Internet]. 2007;28(6):415–8. Available from:
https://www.sciencedirect.com/science/article/pii/S0196070906002638

14. Flynn TR. Principles of Management of Odontogenic Infections. In:
Peterson's principles of oral & maxillofacial surgery. Ontario: BC
Decker; 2004. p. 277–312.

15. Rabie M. Shanti. TRF. Principles of Antimicrobial and Surgical Infection Management. In: Head neck and Orofacial Infections. St. Louis Missouri: Elsevier; 2016. p. 121–40.

16. Rosas LMA, Ballesteros FM, Taborda KNN, Fuentes FAP, Mora JA, Jens CT. Relación anatómico-radiológica de los espacios del cuello. Rev Médica Sanitas [Internet]. 2017 [cited 2022 Feb 25];20(1):40–9. Available from: https://revistas.unisanitas.edu.co/index.php/RMS/article/view/250

17. Matthew E. Lawler. ZP. Imaging for Head, Neck, and Orofacial Infections. In: Head neck and Orofacial Infections. St. Louis Missouri: Elsevier; 2016. p. 103–20.

18. Agarwal AK, Kanekar SG. Submandibular and sublingual spaces: diagnostic imaging and evaluation. Otolaryngol Clin North Am [Internet]. 2012 [cited 2022 Feb 25];45(6):1311–23. Available from: https://www.oto.theclinics.com/article/S0030-6665(12)00119-3/fulltext

19. Sadrameli M, Mupparapu M. Oral and maxillofacial anatomy. Radiol Clin North Am [Internet]. 2018 [cited 2022 Feb 25];56(1):13–29. Available from: https://www.radiologic.theclinics.com/article/S0033-8389(17)30126-4/fulltext

20. Heidegger T. Management of the difficult airway. N Engl J Med [Internet]. 2021;384(19):1836–47. Available from: http://dx.doi.org/10.1056/NEJMra1916801

21.Heim N, Wiedemeyer V, Reich RH, Martini M. The role of C-reactive protein and white blood cell count in the prediction of length of stay in hospital and severity of odontogenic abscess. J Craniomaxillofac Surg

[Internet]. 2018;46(12):2220–6. Available from:
https://www.sciencedirect.com/science/article/pii/S1010518218306140

22.Fu B, McGowan K, Sun JH, Batstone M. Increasing frequency and severity of odontogenic infection requiring hospital admission and surgical management. Br J Oral Maxillofac Surg [Internet]. 2020;58(4):409–15. Available from:
https://www.sciencedirect.com/science/article/pii/S0266435620300140

23. Flynn TR. What are the antibiotics of choice for odontogenic infections, and how long should the treatment course last? Oral Maxillofac Surg Clin North Am [Internet]. 2011 [cited 2022 Feb 25];23(4):519–36, v–vi. Available from:
https://www.oralmaxsurgery.theclinics.com/article/S1042-3699(11)00143-9/fulltext

24. Morton H. Goldberg. RGT. Odontogenic Infections and Deep Fascial Space Infections of Dental Origin. In: Oral and Maxillofacial Infections. Philadelphia, PA: Saunders; 2002. p. 163.

25. Flynn TR. Surgical management of orofacial infections. Atlas Oral Maxillofac Surg Clin North Am [Internet]. 2000 [cited 2022 Mar 1];8(1):77–100. Available from:
https://www.oralmaxsurgeryatlas.theclinics.com/article/S1061-3315(18)30043-X/pdf

26. Bischofberger AS. Drains, Bandages, and External Coaptation. In: Auer JA, Stick J, Kümmerle JM, Prange T, editors. Equine Surgery. St. Louis, Missouri: Elsevier; 2019. p. 280–300.

27. McCarter YS. Laboratory Microbiological Diagnostic Techniques. In: Oral and Maxillofacial Infections. Philadelphia, PA: Saunders; 2002. p. 43–61.

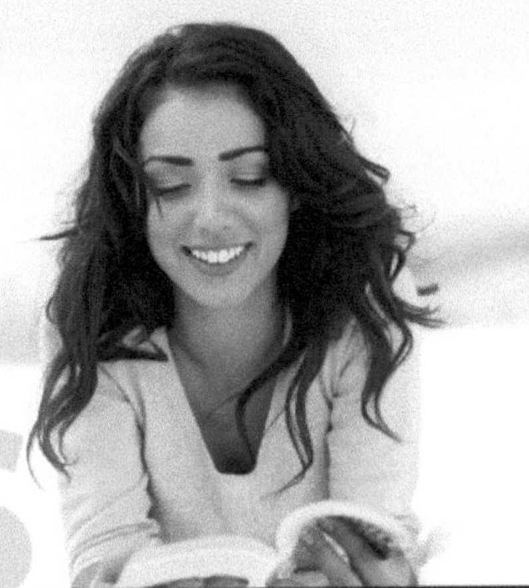

yes
I want morebooks!

Buy your books fast and straightforward online - at one of world's fastest growing online book stores! Environmentally sound due to Print-on-Demand technologies.

Buy your books online at
www.morebooks.shop

Kaufen Sie Ihre Bücher schnell und unkompliziert online – auf einer der am schnellsten wachsenden Buchhandelsplattformen weltweit! Dank Print-On-Demand umwelt- und ressourcenschonend produzi ert.

Bücher schneller online kaufen
www.morebooks.shop

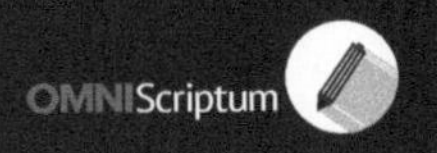

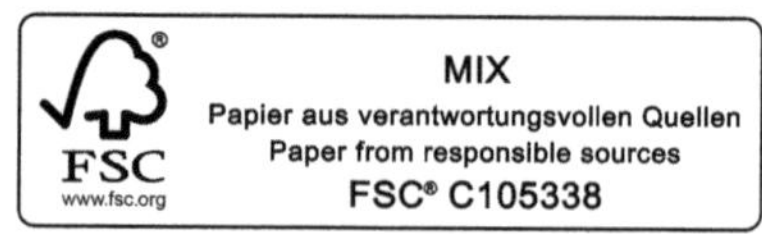

Printed by Books on Demand GmbH, Norderstedt / Germany